STROKE
A Guide for Patient and Family

STROKE
A Guide for Patient and Family

Janice Frye-Pierson, R.N., B.S.N., CNRN

Neurological Nurse Clinician
Department of Neurology
Bowman Gray School of Medicine
Wake Forest University Medical Center
Winston-Salem, North Carolina

James F. Toole, M.D.

Walter C. Teagle Professor of Neurology
Stroke Center Director
Department of Neurology
Bowman Gray School of Medicine
Wake Forest University Medical Center
Winston-Salem, North Carolina

Raven Press 🦅 New York

Raven Press, 1185 Avenue of the Americas, New York, New York 10036

Made in the United States of America

Library of Congress Cataloging-in-Publication Data
Frye-Pierson, Janice.
  Stroke : a guide for patient and family.

  Bibliography: p.
  Includes index.
  1. Cerebrovascular disease—Popular works.
I. Toole, James F., 1925–   . II. Title.
[DNLM: 1. Cerebrovascular Disorders—popular works.
2. Cerebrovascular Disorders—rehabilitation—popular
works. WL 355 F948s]
RC388.5.F78   1987   616.8′1   84-42916
ISBN 0-88167-279-3
ISBN 0-89004-637-9 (pbk.)

The material contained in this volume was submitted as previously unpublished material, except in the instances in which credit has been given to the source from which some of the illustrative material was derived.

Great care has been taken to maintain the accuracy of the information contained in the volume. However, Raven Press cannot be held responsible for errors or for any consequences arising from the use of the information contained herein.

Materials appearing in this book prepared by individuals as part of their official duties as U.S. Government employees are not covered by the above-mentioned copyright.

9 8 7 6 5 4 3 2 1

Dedication

This book is dedicated to patients affected by stroke and their families; to Patricia Neal, who, having had a stroke and making a significant recovery, has done much to promote public awareness on the subject; and to Dr. Lawrence C. McHenry, who gave of his knowledge so freely before his untimely death on February 22, 1985. It is our hope that the battle to decrease the ravages of stroke will be successful.

Preface

Stroke remains one of the least manageable illnesses in the United States despite medical advances aimed at its prevention and treatment. More than 175,000 individuals die of stroke every year, making it the third leading cause of adult death in the United States.

More than half of all stroke patients survive their first stroke, although only about 10% recover completely. The remaining survivors have different degrees of disability, ranging from minimal loss of function to dependency or need for institutionalized care.

The possibility of stroke in ourselves or a loved one is frightening because no one can predict who the next victim will be or the amount of body function or independence that may be lost. Stroke commonly removes from us things we take for granted—simple activities such as walking, talking, writing, and performing functions necessary for daily living. This book will provide insight into the emotional responses of patient and family to such loss of function and how to cope with them.

The control of function of our motor skills is centered in the brain. The brain is composed of nerve cells that require a constant supply of oxygen and glucose for proper maintenance. Oxygen is taken from the air we breathe and glucose from the food we eat. Both are carried in the blood to the brain. If the brain is deprived of these nutrients for as little as 30 seconds, the cells begin to die and a stroke begins.

If a stroke occurs, the life of each family member can undergo many changes. Often the patient is the wage earner and the resulting loss of income requires other members of the family to find additional employment while struggling to pay mounting medical costs. These costs can be astonishing as payments for hospitalization, doctors, medication, necessary home equipment, and rehabilitative therapy continue to rise. Latest figures estimate stroke care in the United States to be more than $6 billion annually.

One of the most difficult decisions for the stroke patient and his or her family is whether to return the patient home after hospitalization. It is the hope that by doing so all concerned can continue their lives much as they were prior to the stroke.

Home adjustments may be required to make this choice feasible. Doors may need to be widened or ramps built to accommodate wheelchairs. Handrails, special cooking equipment, and shower and toilet seat adjustments are just a few changes needed to help make maneuvering easier for the patient. It may be necessary to rearrange furniture and rooms to facilitate the patient's movements.

The physical, emotional, and financial problems that accompany stroke are often complicated further by a lack of understanding of the disease process itself. If the family understands stroke, its causes and effects, its treatment measures, and ways to aid in rehabilitating the stroke survivor, it can give an essential support to the patient's progress.

It is of utmost importance for the patient to have a family prepared and determined to work together for recovery. Involvement in the patient's care should begin early, since an informed, prepared, and understanding family can offer much support. In fact, the family has been shown to be the patient's most effective support system. Often patients follow instructions more readily when given by family members than when given by medical personnel. It is the constant day-to-day struggle together to reach goals that gives the patient and family strength to continue the fight to conquer stroke.

In clear and straightforward terms, this book familiarizes the patient and family with the physiological, emotional, and practical problems associated with stroke, so that these problems can be anticipated and managed. The material here can be used to supplement discussions with the doctors and other members of the patient's stroke team.

Acknowledgments

This book has been completed with the help of many individuals whom we gratefully acknowledge, particularly Kelley N. Williamson, who prepared the manuscript. The artwork was prepared by the Department of Audio-Visual Resources, Bowman Gray School of Medicine. Specifically, we thank Mr. George Lynch, Annemarie Beery, and David Pounds for their contributions.

The following people have also been helpful: Kathy H. Tincher; Diane Vernon; John Wachtel; Deborah C. McKeithan; Barbara Benge, R.N., B.S.N.; Cathy Nunn, R.N., R.V.T.; Lawrence Myers, B.S., R.D.M.S.; Ann H. Connelly, R.N.; Carla Blue, O.T.R.; Drs. C. Steven Ford, Gary R. Kilgo, David S. Lefkowitz, and Arnold E. Nelson; and the Forsyth County Stroke Club, Winston-Salem, North Carolina.

Contents

Contributors

Nancy Crater, R.N., *Rehabilitation Unit, North Carolina Baptist Hospital, 300 South Hawthorne Road, Winston-Salem, North Carolina 27103*

Barbara Freiberg, L.P.T., *Physical Therapist, Department of Physical Therapy, North Carolina Baptist Hospital, 400 South Hawthorne Road, Winston-Salem, North Carolina 27103*

Ronald L. Mace, AIA, *P.O. Box 30634, Water Garden, Highway 70 West, Raleigh, North Carolina 27622*

Claire Matthews, Ph.D., *Speech-Language Pathologist, Department of Communication Disorders, Room 101, St. Louis University, 3733 West Pine Boulevard, St. Louis, Missouri 63108*

Steven S. Pierson, M.D., *Clinical Instructor of Psychiatry, Department of Psychiatry and Behavioral Medicine, Bowman Gray School of Medicine, 300 South Hawthorne Road, Winston-Salem, North Carolina 27103*

J. Stanwood Till, M.D., *Department of Ophthalmology, Louis Gale Clinic, 1802 Braeburn Drive, Salem, Virginia 24153*

1

Definition, Causes, and Risk Factors

In the past the words stroke, cerebral vascular accident (CVA) and apoplexy were used interchangeably as general descriptions of defects in brain function caused by an interruption of its blood supply. Now we have the means by which to determine the cause, and so these general terms have been replaced by precise definitions: infarction, hemorrhage, and embolism.

In order to understand these terms we must consider the heart, arteries, and veins as well as the brain itself. The heart pumps blood containing oxygen and nutrients through the arterial tubes to cells of the body. Veins carry blood back to the heart. Proper maintenance of this supply is essential to ensure normal functioning of the brain.

CAUSES OF STROKE

The signs and symptoms of a stroke can be so minimal that they are hardly recognizable or so severe that the patient is in a coma or dies. They can be temporary or permanent, depending on the extent of the damage. The major causes are infarction caused by thrombosis or embolism (blockage of an artery by a blood clot or foreign body) and hemorrhage.

Infarction

An infarct is an area of tissue that has "died" because of a lack of oxygen supply to it. This lack is due to the blockage

TABLE 1.   *Causes of stroke in the United States*

Cause	%
Thrombosis	52
Embolism	30
Hemorrhage	
Subarachnoid	6
Intracerebral	10
Epidural and subdural	2

caused by a blood clot or buildup within the artery. Most strokes are due to infarction caused by the progressive narrowing or total blockage of arteries due to formation of a blood clot within the artery (Table 1). Thus the inside of the artery (the lumen) becomes so narrow the blood flow becomes blocked.

There are numerous reasons for this narrowing. Among them are thickening of the blood due to an increase in red blood cells, hardening of the arteries (arteriosclerosis), cholesterol and fatty deposits in the artery wall (atherosclerosis), and inflammation of the arteries (arteritis) and veins (phlebitis).

Another cause of stroke, which also results in blockage of blood flow, is embolism. An embolus, usually but not always, is a blood clot or a piece of cholesterol and fat deposit (plaque) that may lodge in arteries too small for it to pass through. It then prevents blood from reaching areas beyond the obstruction, resulting in ischemia, or infarction, of the segment of brain supplied by that artery.

The heart is a common source of emboli. Heart attacks (myocardial infarctions) and irregularities in heartbeat rate and rhythm (atrial fibrillation) are conditions that decrease the power of the heart, thereby decreasing blood flow to the brain. These conditions then encourage the formation of clots, which are potential emboli. Symptoms usually occur suddenly, during either rest or activity.

Hemorrhage

Hemorrhage into the brain, mainly due to uncontrolled high blood pressure, is a major cause of stroke. In this condition the walls of the artery become thicker and less elastic during episodes of high blood pressure. The forceful jet of blood through a damaged artery may cause the vessel to rupture, with the result that blood subsequently flows into the brain. Cerebral hemorrhage, as it is commonly called, is considered the most serious and deadly form of stroke.

Sixteen percent of all strokes are due to hemorrhage of some type. Generally there is a sudden onset of defective functioning, as a headache, stiff neck, nausea and vomiting, often followed by unconsciousness. Individuals who do not lose consciousness generally have a better outlook, and those who become comatose usually die.

Subarachnoid Hemorrhage and Aneurysm

Hemorrhage or excessive bleeding may also occur as a result of a ruptured aneurysm. An aneurysm develops from an abnormality in the wall of the artery that is present at birth. The arterial wall lacks a layer of smooth muscle and elastic tissue and subsequently becomes weak. This weakened area eventually stretches and enlarges to form a ballooning in the wall, referred to as an aneurysm.

Aneurysms are not dangerous unless they rupture or burst. Often the aneurysm is approachable by surgery and can be clamped off from the artery, thereby preventing the possibility of bleeding.

If the aneurysm does rupture, however, hemorrhage results. The blood can then seep under a thin membrane that covers the brain into the subarachnoid space. This condition is referred to as a subarachnoid hemorrhage. This type of hemorrhage can occur at any age but is more commonly seen during the forties and fifties.

Subdural Hemorrhage

Hemorrhage that occurs under the outer hard covering (dura) of the brain is referred to as a subdural hemorrhage or hematoma. Usually this type of hemorrhage results from an injury to the brain caused by the head striking an immovable object. This trauma causes the brain to move in such a manner that the blood vessels are torn, swelling occurs, and a clot is formed. The clot may be removed by drilling a hole in the skull and withdrawing the blood.

Epidural Hemorrhage

An epidural hemorrhage occurs above the outer hard covering of the brain—between this covering and the skull. This type of hemorrhage usually results from a blow to the side of the head that causes damage to arteries and to the surface of the outer covering of the brain. Blood seeps between the layer covering the brain and the brain itself exerts pressure on it. Symptoms from an epidural hemorrhage appear more quickly than those from a subdural hemorrhage. Treatment is the same for both, however: prompt removal of the clot.

Arteriovenous Malformations

An arteriovenous malformation (AVM) is an abnormality of the blood vessels in the brain. These vessels do not differentiate into arteries, veins, and capillaries after birth but instead form a tangle of vessels. Blood then flows directly from the arteries to the veins without properly nourishing the area of the brain as intended. As the veins receive blood that is under the pressure of the arteries, they are likely to rupture and bleed into the brain. Rupture generally occurs in about one-half of AVM patients and takes place between the ages of 20 and 30. These individuals may experience a convulsion as the initial symptom.

Other Causes

There are other conditions that contribute to brain hemorrhage. Specific conditions such as leukemia, Hodgkin's disease, sickle cell anemia, and hemophilia are a few disorders that can interfere with the clotting of blood and thereby cause hemorrhage.

Patients taking excessive amounts of blood-thinning medications are also susceptible to hemorrhage. Therefore it is essential that a prescribed plan be followed and blood be examined periodically to determine if the correct dosage is being given.

It has been found that diet pills and other drugs containing phenylpropanolamine hydrochloride can contribute to stroke by causing increases in blood pressure. It is essential that individuals taking this type of pill, as with all types of medication, be familiar with the warning label and take only as recommended.

RISK FACTORS

Some situations increase the risk of having a stroke. Some can be avoided, and others cannot. Being aware of these risks is important not only to the patient but to the family as well. It is essential that the patient and family attempt to decrease the risk situation in order to prevent or avoid the first or another stroke from occurring. Recognized risk factors are listed in Table 2.

Controllable Factors

High blood pressure (hypertension) is the most common risk factor. Blood pressure is the force of the blood as it is pumped from the heart through the arteries. There are two aspects of the blood pressure that are measured. The first measurement is obtained when the heart is working its hardest to pump the

TABLE 2. *Controllable and noncontrollable risk factors for stroke*

Controllable factors	Noncontrollable factors
High blood pressure	Age
Diabetes mellitus	Sex
High cholesterol and blood fats	Race
Heart disease	Hereditary factors
Transient ischemic attacks (TIAs)	
Oral contraceptives	
Increased blood viscosity (thick blood)	
Smoking	
Obesity	

blood (systolic pressure); the second is obtained when the heart is relaxed (diastolic pressure). Blood pressure is reported in millimeters of mercury (mm Hg). A normal blood pressure is equal to or below 140/90 mm Hg, while a sustained pressure equal to or greater than 160/95 mm Hg is considered high. Blood pressure values between these normal and high values are termed borderline. Blood pressures constantly change, therefore pressures must be taken routinely and if a prolonged elevation is noted, a diagnosis of high blood pressure (hypertension) is made.

Blood pressure can become abnormally elevated and push blood through the arteries at a force and rate higher than normal, causing damage to the walls of the blood vessel. Damage increases as the arteries become hardened and narrowed over a period of time. Moreover, the increased pressure can force a piece of plaque loose or contribute to the rupture of an aneurysm, as discussed earlier.

There are at least 23 million and perhaps as many as 40 million people in the United States whose usual blood pressure is more than 140/90 mm Hg. These individuals are at greatly increased risk of stroke, heart disease, and kidney failure. The shocking fact is that about one-third do not even know that they have a problem because high blood pressure (hypertension) is a silent disease, producing no symptoms until it has damaged the eyes, heart, or kidneys. It is all the more shocking because it has been proved that treatment of hypertension dramatically reduces such complications as heart failure, strokes, blindness, and kidney failure. The better the control of the hypertension, the longer one lives comfortably. The importance of detecting high blood pressure is that it can usually be controlled successfully by medication. Yet no more than one-eighth of all hypertensive persons are adequately controlled because of a variety of problems, including cost of medicine or reluctance to take pills.

Therefore periodic checks should be done to ensure a normal pressure. Note that just because the blood pressure is normal at one time, it does not mean it will be the next. It is essential that the individual follow diet and medication instructions that are aimed at reducing the elevated blood pressure. Decreasing sodium intake is helpful. Ham, cheese, sausage, and foods containing self-rising flour have a high amount of salt in them. Canned vegetables and convenience foods also contain a high amount of sodium and should be replaced with fresh vegetables. Spices may be used instead of salt to flavor foods.

Individuals with *diabetes mellitus* are also at risk for having a stroke. With diabetes, there is an excessive level of a simple sugar (glucose) found in the blood because of the body's inability to metabolize glucose properly. Over a period of time, diabetes causes damage to blood vessels, making the individual more susceptible to hardening of the arteries (arteriosclerosis). As arteriosclerosis continues to develop, blood flow through the artery becomes increasingly difficult. This process may eventually restrict blood flow altogether.

The symptoms of diabetes mellitus are elevated blood glucose, glucose noted in the urine, excessive urination, increased thirst, increased appetite, and generalized weakness. Those who are most susceptible to developing diabetes have some of the same characteristics as many stroke patients. Generally, individuals who are significantly overweight, are over 40 years of age, and have a history of diabetes in their families are prone to develop this condition.

There is no known cure for diabetes, but there are effective treatment measures. The choice of treatment depends on many factors, including the severity of the disease, the patient's age, and the symptoms. Diet and exercise alone are often effective in managing diabetes. However, medication given as a pill or by injection may be needed once or twice a day. It is essential that diabetes be managed properly, not only to decrease one's risk for stroke but also to prevent other complications that may arise as a result of the disease.

There are certain types of dietary cholesterols and fats that the body utilizes to provide energy, enabling cells to function effectively. However, some of the cholesterol and fat products cannot be broken down and used properly. Thus a diet high in *cholesterol and fats* (*lipids*) can promote atherosclerosis. This process may eventually cause plaque to build up on the artery wall, so that blood cannot flow through the artery. The plaque may also break off and function in the same way a blood clot does—by lodging in a small area and preventing blood flow beyond that point. Therefore following a diet low in cholesterol and fats aids in preventing atherosclerosis.

Foods to avoid that are high in cholesterol are milk, butter, margarine, cream, eggs, cheese, meat, and lard. Foods that contain a small amount of cholesterol are vegetables, fruit, skimmed milk, cottage cheese, yogurt, and oils (such as corn, vegetable, and olive oil).

Cardiac factors such as heart attack (myocardial infarction) and an abnormal heart beat rate and rhythm (atrial fibrillation) also increase one's risk for stroke. When the power of the pump (heart) is decreased, there is decreased blood flow to the brain. Also remember that the heart is a major source of blood clots (emboli), which can lodge in an area too small for them to pass on the way to the brain. The brain is then deprived of oxygen and nutrients, which causes death of the tissue (infarction).

A major risk factor for stroke is a *transient ischemic attack* (TIA). TIAs are episodes of neurological deficits usually lasting 5 to 30 minutes or longer, after which the symptoms resolve, returning the affected individual to his previous state. Individuals usually have a complete recovery with no detectable deficits after 24 hours. If a deficit is noted after that time, the patient has suffered a stroke, not a TIA.

Transient ischemic attacks are commonly thought to be warning signs that resolve before a stroke occurs. A TIA has the same importance as chest pain: Both warn the physician that something more urgent and extreme may occur if proper therapy is not begun. As many as one-third of individuals experiencing TIAs go on to have a stroke. Due to the importance of this subject, it is discussed in more detail in a later chapter.

Women who are pregnant or taking *oral contraceptives* (birth control pills) are at high risk for stroke. Blood can thicken under these conditions, largely due to an increase in hormone levels. Furthermore, women who experience migraine headaches *and* take a birth control pill have an increased susceptibility to stroke. The risk is further increased if the woman smokes as well. The increased risk is due to the combined effects of spasm of arteries (seen with migraine headaches and smoking) and thickened blood (noted with the pill).

It is important that women who take oral contraceptives and smoke or experience migraine headaches consider whether oral contraception is the best choice of birth control for them. Often another form should be selected in order to decrease the risk of stroke.

Individuals with *thick blood* are also at risk for stroke. An overproduction of red blood cells with a subsequent increase in hematocrit (ratio of red blood cells to fluid content of the blood) may occur. Thus the blood becomes thick and sludges, thereby plugging small blood vessels. Often this condition requires a phlebotomy to lower the amount of red blood cells: With phlebotomy a recommended amount of blood is removed from the patient over a period of days. (The fluid portion is replaced by natural means faster than the cells, resulting in "thinner" blood.)

Smoking has not been proved conclusively to be a primary risk factor for stroke but is a highly suspected one. However, smoking causes spasm of arteries and thus may create difficulty in blood flow. Furthermore, smoking is a known risk factor for heart disease, and can cause a stroke secondary to the heart problem. Therefore individuals should refrain from smoking to decrease their risks for stroke and heart disease.

Three times as many strokes occur among men who are heavy smokers as in nonsmokers. Among those who stop smoking completely, there is an obvious decrease in the death rate for heart disease during the first year. Yet when the rate of previous smokers is compared to that of nonsmokers, results show it takes 10 years or more to reduce the death rate of previous smokers to that of nonsmokers. Thus the sooner one stops smoking, the better his overall health will be.

It is not easy to stop smoking. Some individuals go "cold turkey," whereas others attempt it gradually. Specific helpful suggestions (if difficult) are to smoke filter cigarettes that are low in tar and nicotine; attempt to lower the number of cigarettes smoked daily; try not to inhale; and do switch from cigarettes to a pipe or cigars. Pipe smoking keeps one from inhaling as much of the offending substances. However, when using a pipe use small amounts of tobacco in order not to equal the effect obtained from smoking cigarettes.

Obesity is also suspected to increase the risk for stroke. Often overweight individuals eat a diet high in fats and cholesterol, sugar, and salt, all of which contribute to atherosclerosis, diabetes, and high blood pressure. Excess weight can cause additional stress on the heart as well. Therefore a sensible diet along with a moderate amount of exercise is an effective way to stay in shape. Walking has been proved to be an efficient form of exercise, not only for correcting obesity but for reducing other risk factors as well.

Usually people are at their ideal weight between the ages of 18 and 21. Most generally know if they are overweight by comparing their weights then and now. However, some people have had to deal with being overweight since childhood. There are many tables and methods in use to help determine ideal weight. A simple method is to bend forward and measure an area of skin below the ribs. If it measures an inch or more, it is an indication of being overweight. A physician may be able to supply tables of ideal weights.

Controlling these risk factors is an effective way to prevent stroke or a recurrence. In review, specific guidelines are to maintain one's blood pressure at or below 140/90 mm Hg, keep cholesterol levels below 210 mg/dl for men and 180 mg/dl for women, do not smoke, maintain blood glucose levels below 120 mg/dl, and attempt to keep body weight within an ideal range.

Noncontrollable Factors

Stroke has no boundaries as to *age, race, or sex*. Thus anyone can be affected. Men appear to have a higher incidence of stroke in their earlier years than women. Some experts believe it may be due to the added protection given women by female hormones. Interestingly, however, the incidence of stroke in women after menopause is equal to that in men of the same age. Most of the individuals who experience hemorrhage are Black, probably because of their increased incidence of high blood pressure. It is unknown why Blacks have an increased incidence of high blood pressure.

The extent to which *inherited factors* contribute to stroke is not known. However, a correlation does appear to exist. It is possible, however, that increased stress and poor dietary patterns (environmental factors) contribute, making one more susceptible to stroke.

2

Anatomy

The brain is located within the skull, which along with the hair and scalp, protects the brain from injury. The brain is so delicate and its function so easily disturbed that it is suspended in fluid for even more protection. The spinal cord is an extension of the brain and lies within the vertebrae of the spine. The brain is composed of about 60 billion cells and the connections between them. When it is working properly and the connections are made, it results in thinking and remembering; emotional reactions such as anger, happiness, sadness; the activities that protect the body (such as the need to eat and sleep, and the regulation of such functions as blood pressure, hunger, bowel activity, and breathing); and finally the regulation of all of our behavior, including reproductive activities. Although it is not within the scope of this book to describe brain function, one cannot consider stroke and its treatment without understanding how the brain works.

COMPOSITION OF THE BRAIN

The brain is composed of cells that interrelate with each other through hair-like tentacles (which under a microscope look almost like roots of a plant or perhaps a jellyfish). These many extensions touch other cells, forming a means of communication via electrical messages and by minute amounts of secretions, which become chemical messengers.

In order to operate properly, the 60 billion cells that form the human brain must have an uninterrupted supply of glucose (fuel) and oxygen with which to keep the metabolism of the cells functioning. These cells do not use protein or fat for their metabolic activities—only sugar in the form of glucose, of which it utilizes 150 grams (approximately 1 cup full) daily along with 72 liters of oxygen (about a bathtub full). Because the brain cannot store these substances it can function for only a few minutes if they are reduced below critical levels. The lungs breathe in air containing oxygen, which is transferred to the arterial blood and pumped to the brain by the heart through the major arteries. The veins remove waste products, principally carbon dioxide, acid metabolites, and heat from the brain, transporting it back to the heart where it can be excreted through the lungs or the kidneys.

BLOOD SUPPLY TO THE BRAIN

Each time the heart beats it thrusts about 70 milliliters (ml) of blood into the aorta of which 10 to 15 ml goes to the brain. The heart beats about 70 times a minute and sends 700 to 1,000 ml of blood to the brain each minute, or almost 1,440 liters (1,500 quarts) every 24 hours. Because the brain weighs about 1,500 grams the blood flow allocated to it is in the range of 50 ml per 100 grams per minute.

Each cerebral hemisphere has its own carotid artery that goes up through the neck, behind the angle of the jaw, and penetrates the bones at the base of the skull to enter the cranial cavity (Fig. 1). The carotid artery can be felt beside the trachea in the neck. It should not be pressed hard because in some people sensitivity of this artery is such that blockage of the artery makes them faint either because of a lack of blood supply or a reflex called the carotid sinus reflex. The common carotid artery divides into two branches: the external carotid artery, which supplies the face and structures outside the skull, and the internal carotid artery, which supplies the eye and the brain. The internal carotid artery gives off several major branches, the blockage of any one of which can result

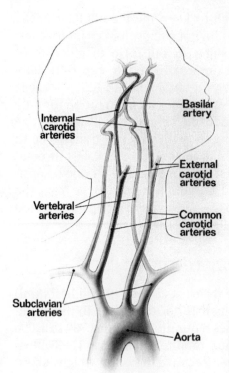

Internal carotid arteries

Basilar artery

External carotid arteries

Vertebral arteries

Common carotid arteries

Subclavian arteries

Aorta

FIG. 1. The brain is supplied with blood flowing from the heart through the carotid and vertebral arteries.

in a stroke. The first of these is the artery to the eye (the ophthalmic artery). Above this branch several other branches supply the brain's temporal lobes, frontal lobes, and parts of the parietal lobes.

The back of the brain receives its blood from the vertebral and basilar arteries (Fig. 1). This system arises from the subclavian arteries, which also supply blood to the arms. The vertebral arteries travel to the head through the bony canal in the neck and into the skull through the large opening that contains the spinal cord. The two arteries then join to form the basilar artery. This artery provides nourishment for the inner ear, the brainstem, and the cerebellum, about which there is more later.

Therefore the brain is dependent on four arteries for its supply of blood and nutrition. Theoretically, occlusion or blockage of any one of those arteries would leave a vital area of the brain without blood supply. Nature has, however, provided magnificent protection for this supply: the circle of Willis, named for the man who first described it. This circle lies at the base of the brain and connects all four arteries so that when one is blocked blood can travel from the other three to take over the area that is normally supplied by the blocked artery. There are many instances in which people have had one, two, and sometimes three arteries blocked without developing any abnormalities as a result. In these cases the blood supply has been taken over by the collateral arteries.

Some of the major sources of the interconnections between arteries in addition to the circle of Willis are through the eye, between the external and internal carotid arteries, and through the muscles of the neck. As a group, these rich interconnections protect the brain by allowing alternate routes that can bypass obstructions in any of the main arteries that supply the brain. For example, obstruction of the internal carotid artery in the neck may be bypassed by external carotid branches that flow through the eye and rejoin the internal carotid artery distal to the obstruction. Within the brain the blood vessels distribute blood through vessels of decreasing size.

AREAS OF THE BRAIN

The brain is divided into right and left cerebral hemispheres, the brainstem, and the cerebellum. These structures connect with the outside world by nerves that conduct electrical and chemical messages between the brain and spinal cord and the sense organs and muscles of the body. The functions of the brain can be distinguished from one another. For example, speech is located in only one hemisphere, which is usually the left side of the brain, whereas memory is located in both temporal lobes, and vision in both occipital lobes (Fig. 2). Many

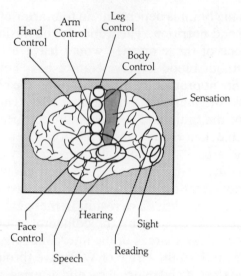

FIG. 2. Control zones of the brain. (Redrawn by permission of the American Heart Association, Inc. In: *Strokes—A Guide for the Family.* American Heart Association, 1981.)

of the aspects of creativity and innovation come from the frontal lobes.

To understand how the system works, consider how to drive an automobile. It requires inputs from vision, hearing, balance, touch, memory, and the capacity to react quickly to changing situations as when using the steering wheel or applying the accelerator or brakes. Remember how difficult it was when you first learned to drive a car and how nervous and anxious you were? Each movement had to be performed consciously, and you were afraid you might forget one of them and cause an accident. You were alert and thinking about each action. You were learning to use several functions of the brain at once in order to learn a new skill. This functioning is one of the major aspects of the brain—the capacity to learn new tasks and to recall the information when it is needed.

First you developed the understanding of what driving is by

watching others with your eyes. This information was received in the occipital lobes of the brain as electrical impulses and then stored in the parietal lobes just in front. When you first practiced driving you used sight and sound to guide you on the road, the temporal lobes to remember where to go, and the frontal lobes to give you insight and judgment as to why you are going.

CAPACITIES OF THE BRAIN

The human has the most advanced brain of all the species and as a consequence has the capacity to adapt to new situations. In this regard, therefore, once having learned to drive you could go over highways to new places, follow road maps, and enjoy the scenery without even thinking of the actual work of driving.

Take another example—speaking and reading. These abilities are found only in humans; no other animal species has acquired them. Babies learn to speak by imitating their elders and mouthing sounds. It requires altering velocity and causing vibration in the air that is coming out of the lungs. It is done by controlling the positions of the vocal cords, tongue, and lips with appropriate muscles, causing the air to vibrate at different frequencies and tones, and interrupting the flow of air by periods of silence. Air then moves into the listener's ear, causing the eardrums to vibrate in response. The mechanical energy changes to electricity, which travels through the auditory nerves to the brain. Both the sender who is speaking and the receiver who is listening understand the code; it is called language. There are hundreds of languages on the earth, and it is only by mutual consent that a certain sound means a certain object or idea. Children learn the language of their parents by associating sounds with objects, actions, and ideas. Later the child learns to read and translates symbols he can see on paper into the sounds he has already learned. For example, if he learns to like the taste of a banana and learns the sound of the word, later he can be taught to read *b-a-n-a-n-a* printed on a page. He remembers it from the store of information in his brain, and he can visualize what it looks like and how it tastes.

For most people, reading a word conjures up a visual image of what has been seen in the past. As the facility to read increases, however, one can become detached from the individual words and read without conscious thinking just as one can drive automatically. Writing is the manual expression of reading accomplished by learning to form the symbols that enable one to express by written symbols what one is thinking in one's brain.

As children grow, they improve their social behavior and are taught insight and judgment so that they do not make dangerous or foolish mistakes, and they learn social responsibility for themselves and for others. During their exploratory phase children must be watched constantly, otherwise they run into the street, for example, or put their hands in dangerous places; with the passage of time and teaching by the parents, however, they do it less and less frequently until by the time they are "mature" they may no longer do foolish things. To return for a moment to the example of the person learning to drive, we all know that in the beginning one is extremely cautious, worried about damaging the car or having an accident. Fear is a function of survival that is located in the upper part of the brainstem. As one becomes more skilled, this caution disappears and the person who has now had 1 or 2 years of driving may well become overconfident, ignore dangers, and even drive recklessly. The most dangerous ages for driving are in the teens and early twenties, at a time when youths are theoretically mature but still at a transitional age when child-like activities can interfere with their social behavior. Alcohol is a particular problem in this group because it removes the functions of the part of brain that keeps one cautious and responsible. Speaking, reading, writing, and judgment are called higher cortical functions.

In addition to these higher functions, the two hemispheres control the motor functions of the four limbs. The left brain controls the right side of the body so that when a person combs his hair with his right hand, the left brain is commanding the movement. In other activities that use both arms or both legs, as riding a bicycle, both sides of the body must be working simultaneously or alternately, so that the two hemispheres must cooperate with each other, and there must be transfer and close coordination and timing between the two sides.

Throughout one's adult life all of these activities are done without thought: They have become automatic movements. As time goes on, brain activity may begin to diminish, and at times Alzheimer's disease or a stroke destroys functions that have been present during mature years. In these cases, the capacity to perform activities is lost or vastly reduced. It is distressing for everyone, including the individual who is affected, to realize that the functions one could perform with ease have now become impossible. How humiliating it must be for the person with a neurological disorder who had always been able to control his bowel and bladder and to take care of all of his hygiene needs to become dependent on somebody else for these activities.

DISRUPTION OF BRAIN FUNCTIONS

Have you ever been to the circus and watched the trapeze artists and the tightrope walkers perform and wonder how they keep their balance and have such a marvelous sense of precision and timing? These functions are controlled by the cerebellum. Signs of disease of the cerebellum are an unsteady gait and lack of coordination. People commonly speak of the disturbed walking seen with cerebellar disease as a "drunken gait."

All of these functions are extinguished within 30 seconds if the brain does not receive its proper supply of blood, which has been carrying oxygen and glucose to the brain cells. The blood flowing to the brain goes through a series of muscular tubes called arteries that have a smooth inner lining so that the blood does not clot or adhere to it. The muscles can constrict and make tubes smaller or larger. The blood is pumped out of the heart with each beat; thus the heart is a pump that forces blood containing oxygen from the lungs into the muscular tubes (arteries), some of which carry the blood up through the neck into the skull and then to the brain.

Feel your neck just above the collar bone. Can you feel the artery pulsing? Further up in the neck near the angle of the jaw is the area where the carotid artery divides into a bridge that supplies the muscles and skin of the face (the external carotid artery) and another bridge that goes straight up to the brain (the internal carotid artery). This critical area is where most strokes start. The spot where the artery divides is called a bifurcation, and for some reason, as yet unknown to scientists, arteriosclerotic plaques (hardened areas) tend to aggregate there. In so doing, they plug the artery with debris that may break off and be carried by the blood to the brain, causing an embolism. Alternatively, the artery itself may become totally plugged, causing an occlusion or thrombosis.

3

Symptoms, Signs, and Syndromes

There are several ways to think about stroke. The first is to look at it in terms of the cause; another is according to the location of the damage; and a third is concerned with the size of the lesion. Each of these factors affects how the stroke begins, how long it lasts, and the degree of recovery there will be.

Another way in which a stroke can be classified is by the symptoms it causes. In some cases the usual symptoms seen with stroke last only a short period of time—minutes to hours—and then resolve without evidence of ever having occurred. These episodes are known as transient ischemic attacks (TIAs). A typical example is discussed below.

Mr. P. had completed another busy day at the office. He had never thought that being an assistant vice-president would mean so much added responsibility. Yet being a compulsive type, he knew that he could handle just about anything—even if it meant longer and more stressful hours.

Now that the day was over, Mr. P. was headed for his usual workout on the racquetball court. He was proud that at 48 years of age he offered good competition even to younger players. Along with trying to stay in shape, he thought that most of his success was due to his determination to win. Being best meant everything to him.

This particular day, Mr. P. was not at his best, despite his efforts. His partner, a long time friend, was ahead and was quite a challenge for him. Maybe he was not concentrating as he should. After all, he was worried about the merger he had been trying to complete with a major corporation.

Suddenly, Mr. P. felt a sharp pain in his chest. He had experienced it before and thought it to be indigestion. Maybe he should not have eaten a burger and fries for lunch while working at his desk. Usually, he stayed away from fried foods, but lately work had not allowed enough time for a more balanced diet.

The game continued, and Mr. P. was determined to conquer the indigestion, as well as his opponent. He gave a hard swing and immediately lost control and dropped the racquet. His arm had no strength! His friend rushed over to see what had happened. As Mr. P. began to explain, he noticed that his tongue felt thick and his speech was slurred. He decided to take his friend's suggestion and go to the locker room to rest.

Approximately 5 minutes passed and Mr. P.'s arm was still weak and his speech had not improved. Furthermore, his friend told him that his mouth was drooping on the right side. He decided that he should go to the hospital to find out what was happening. His partner was more than willing to take him.

On the way there, he noticed that his arm was slowly getting strength back. When talking to the emergency room personnel, he also noticed that his speech sounded better. By the time he was seen by a nurse he had improved significantly.

Mr. P. was seen by a physician approximately an hour after he had dropped his racquet. By then his strength had returned to normal. The doctor heard the story from Mr. P. and his friend. He decided to order some tests examining the condition of Mr. P.'s heart and brain. It would also be good to note the blood flow of the arteries from the heart to the brain. The doctor told Mr. P. that he had experienced a transient ischemic attack, commonly referred to as a TIA.

Some individuals experience symptoms from defects that resolve within weeks. These episodes are known as reversible ischemic neurological deficits (RINDs). Recognizing RINDs is important, as beginning proper treatment may prevent a major stroke.

A progressing stroke develops gradually over a period of hours to days. One such case is told here.

Mr. B. decided to go to bed earlier than usual. It was going to be a busy day, as he had much to do. Mr. B.'s grandson, Jimmy, was coming to visit the next day.

Jimmy had accomplished a lot during the past year. He was the first in his family to attend college, and that meant a great deal to Mr. B. Having quit school in the fourth grade to work on the family farm, Mr. B. was proud that his grandson was getting the education he never had. It was even more exciting that Jimmy had received a scholarship for the 4 years he would be studying for an engineering degree. Jimmy's parents were farmers just like Mr. B. had been, and their income depended on a good crop. Thus going to college was not considered something they could normally have afforded for Jimmy.

Upon awakening, Mr. B. noticed a tingling feeling in his left hand. He started rubbing his hand, assuming he had slept on it, preventing good circulation, but it did not seem to help.

Mr. B. began fixing breakfast, thinking a good meal helps any problem. He became upset when he dropped the eggs he was holding in his left hand. He could not believe that he had lost his grip until he suddenly realized that his arm and hand had become weak.

As this day was so important to Mr. B., he did not want to jump to conclusions and alarm anyone. He decided that he probably had become too excited about his grandson's visit, and the weakness was the result of a bad case of "nerves." Therefore he decided to go back to bed and try to relax. He was somewhat frightened but thought things would soon be better.

After a short nap, he awoke and realized his arm was still weak. He could barely move it now. As he was now more frightened, he decided to call his daughter and tell her to bring Jimmy the next day. Yet he did not want her to get excited and call the doctor. A visit to the doctor and another bottle of pills was just too much of a strain on Mr. B.'s social security check. He was already taking pills for high blood pressure that were so costly he often did not take them when he was feeling well.

Upon getting out of bed Mr. B. fell and realized that his left leg had now become weak as well. For a few moments he was so scared he did not know what to do.

At this point he knew he must ask for help, and he would have to find a way. Mr. B. began crawling toward the phone in the adjacent hallway using his good arm and leg to pull his body, inch by inch. He managed to jerk the phone down to the floor by pulling on the cord, and he dialed the operator.

Mr. B. told the operator to call for an ambulance and gave her his daughter's number to call. As she was only a mile or so down the road, Mr. B. knew she would be there soon.

Within minutes she arrived and found Mr. B. in the floor, next to the phone. His words were now slurred and his face drawn. The rescue squad arrived next and told them Mr. B. was having a stroke. It seemed impossible to Mr. B. that what had started out hours earlier as tingling in his arm had gone this far.

In some cases stroke can be prevented from progressing further if prompt treatment is given, such as medication to thin the blood (anticoagulants) or perhaps surgery. In some cases the defects that caused the stroke stabilize without improving or progressing. The term given for this condition is a *completed stroke*. At the present time, there is no specific treatment that quickly reverses this situation, but current research suggests that ways will be discovered for the brain cells to regrow or new ones will appear to replace those that have been killed by the stroke. However, this research is still in the early stages and is not yet being applied clinically.

It is important that the patient be observed for any medical complications of stroke and that further problems be prevented. When the patient's condition is stable, attempts to regain function are instituted. We discuss this area below and give tips on how to minimize the effects of stroke in a subsequent chapter.

TRANSIENT ISCHEMIC ATTACKS

The warning signs of a stroke need to be understood. A TIA is an episode of neurological deficit that indicates a loss of blood flow to the brain. The episode may last 5 minutes to 24 hours. The difference between a TIA and a stroke is that with a TIA the symptoms are resolved in 24 hours without evidence of ever being present. If the defect continues after that, a stroke has occurred.

If one has a TIA, this warning makes him 16 times more likely to have a stroke in the near future. Furthermore, there is a much greater risk of having a stroke within the first year following a TIA. Therefore this warning attack is an emergency and requires rapid evaluation of the patient to prevent occurrence of a subsequent stroke.

An important aspect when evaluating an individual suspected of having a TIA is the history of the attack. Often by the time a patient is seen by medical personnel the symptoms have resolved. Thus it is essential that the person and others observing the event be able to give as accurate a description as possible of the episode(s). Being aware of the symptoms and their duration is helpful to the physician.

It is essential to be familiar with the symptoms that suggest a TIA, which can persist and become a stroke. These symptoms can indicate which areas of the brain are experiencing difficulty with blood flow. (Refer to Fig. 1 in Chap. 2, which shows the areas that perform particular functions.)

As mentioned earlier there are four major arteries that bring blood from the heart to the brain. The carotid and vertebral arteries travel up the front (anterior) portion of each side of the neck and divide into the internal and external branches. Only the internal carotid artery normally supplies the brain.

Carotid Artery Problems

Symptoms accounting for a TIA in the carotid distribution are discussed in the following sections.

Weakness and Sensory Problems

Motor deficits and loss of sensation are commonly seen as symptoms of TIAs in the carotid system. In most individuals the right hemisphere of the brain controls the left side and vice versa. Thus an individual experiencing difficulty with blood flow to the right side of the brain may note weakness and/or numbness on the left side of the body. The terms "hemiparesis" or "hemiplegia" are often used to describe weakness on one side of the body ("hemi" meaning half). Hemisensory loss refers to an inability to note sensation on the opposite side from the involvement in the brain.

Speech and Language Problems

Speech and language difficulties are also seen as symptoms of insufficient blood in the carotid system. Dysarthria or slurred speech is most commonly seen as a symptom that represents a disturbance of blood flow in the vertebrobasilar system. However, weakness of facial muscles (sometimes seen with carotid artery disease) can result, making speech so difficult that slurring occurs.

Aphasia is the term used to describe the inability to understand and use the symbols of language, both spoken and written. It can involve either a motor or a sensory component.

A speech deficit due to damage to the motor strip of the brain results in the individual understanding what is being said to him, but he has difficulty writing legibly or speaking fluently (expressive aphasia).

An individual experiencing a speech deficit with involvement along the sensory strip notes an inability to understand what is said to him, even though his speech may be fluent (receptive aphasia). Often his speech is gibberish and makes little sense, which may be due to a lack of understanding of what he wants to communicate.

Ninety-nine percent of right-handed individuals and 60% of left-handed individuals have their speech center located in the left hemisphere (side) of their brain. This situation is often referred to as being left hemisphere dominant. Thus disturbance of blood flow to the left hemisphere may present speech problems more often in these individuals than in those with right hemisphere dominance.

Vision Problems

Vision problems that result from disease in the carotid arteries involve either half or all of the visual field. One type of problem the patient may experience is a sudden, fleeting loss of vision in an entire eye, referred to as amaurosis fugax. Often when taking the history of a patient who has had one of these episodes, it is common for him to describe the incident as if a shade was pulled up or down over his eye.

The cause for this temporary blindness in an eye is often due to the lodging of an blood clot (embolus) in an artery going to the eye. Blood flow is thus interrupted, and blindness occurs. This condition is temporary, as the clot eventually breaks up and allows blood to resume its normal flow pattern. Another factor that may contribute to this condition is narrowing of the artery, which reduces the blood flow to the eye.

Another visual complaint is the loss of one-half of the visual

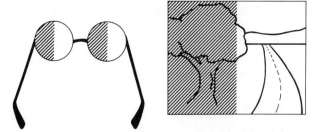

FIG. 3. The patient with homonymous hemianopsia loses half of his field of vision in each eye and fails to recognize entire objects.

field on the outer (temporal) side of one eye and one-half of the field on the inner (nasal) side of the other eye, referred to as homonymous hemianopsia. This visual defect can be appreciated by blocking out half the nasal and corresponding temporal side of a pair of glasses. Often patients with this problem are unaware it exists until they do something that requires them to look to one side and they discover their inability to see properly. A common example is not recognizing an approaching object when turning to back out of an area while driving because of the loss of that visual field (Fig. 3).

Vertebral Artery Problems

The vertebral arteries travel to the brain through the vertebral column in the neck. Upon entering the skull, they form the basilar artery and are often referred to as the vertebrobasilar system. This system is responsible for supplying blood to the brainstem, cerebellum, and occipital portion of the brain.

It is usually possible to distinguish the carotid (anterior) circulation TIAs from the vertebrobasilar (posterior) circulation TIAs. Symptoms accounting for a TIA in the vertebrobasilar distribution are discussed in the following sections.

Weakness and Sensory Problems

Motor and sensory deficits also occur in the vertebrobasilar distribution. However, rather than one side being affected, more often both arms or legs (or both) are involved. In some situations there is a shifting of these symptoms: first one extremity is involved, then another.

Speech Problems

Slurred speech (dysarthria) is more commonly noted here than with carotid disease, as discussed earlier. This problem is due to the interruption of blood to the cranial nerves that control the muscles necessary for speech, located in the vertebrobasilar distribution.

Vision Problems

Visual disturbances are also symptoms of TIAs in this distribution. Double vision and loss of vision in a particular field, described earlier, are common visual complaints.

Drop Attacks

Drop attacks may occur when there is ischemia (lack of blood) to the area of the brain supplied by this arterial system. Often these attacks occur when the vertebral arteries are kinked, as in the neck upon turning the head.

These episodes are described as a loss of strength in the lower extremities, causing one to fall to the floor without losing consciousness. Thus it is not as if one fainted or had a seizure, as consciousness is maintained. Often a patient who has experienced a drop attack gives a history of looking up or reaching for something, whereupon he suddenly fell to the floor while maintaining consciousness.

Subclavian Steal Syndrome

A syndrome that generally exhibits vertebrobasilar symptoms is that of the subclavian steal syndrome. More commonly the left subclavian artery is involved. The cause is attributed to narrowing of the subclavian artery close to the vertebral artery. Thus blood must travel a different route, through the opposite vertebral artery, in order to supply blood to areas normally supplied by the subclavian artery.

There are certain features that aid in determining if one has this syndrome. A delayed and weakened-to-absent radial pulse along with a difference in blood pressure in both arms are common signs. This delay and diminished flow occurs because of the different route blood must take to supply the areas unable to be reached through the narrowed subclavian artery, as discussed earlier.

The presence of a murmur (bruit) at the involved subclavian artery is another feature of this syndrome. The bruit indicates a disturbance in blood flow due to plaque buildup of the artery wall, which contributes to stenosis.

Exercising the involved limb produces symptoms. So long as the arm does not receive the amount of blood necessary for its functioning, neurological deficits occur. More commonly there is dizziness along with weakness and numbness of the involved extremity.

Confirmation that this syndrome is present, despite the clinical signs and symptoms, depends on angiography. This test consists in a radiopaque dye being injected into the arteries, which then demonstrates the blockage and backward flow on x-ray films.

TRANSIENT GLOBAL AMNESIA

C.B., a 57-year-old, right-handed, white male college professor, was brought to the emergency room by his wife after experiencing a loss of memory for approximately 4 hours (11:00 a.m. to 3:30 p.m.).

His wife saw him during the episode of amnesia. She stated that he came home at about noon and told her that he had some errands to do and left the house again. She did not think that his behavior was unusual or inappropriate. She did state, however, that he had awakened that morning with a headache and told her that he still had the headache when she questioned him about it at lunch.

At around 3:30 p.m. that afternoon, he came to his "senses" and found himself sitting alone in his car. He remembered getting out of his car and asking someone the date and time. He then drove home but remained somewhat confused, as he could not explain the directions he took to get to his house.

After relating the story to his wife and realizing that he had not remembered anything since leaving school around 11:00 a.m., Mrs. B. decided to take her husband to the nearby emergency room. There they were told that Mr. B. had experienced an episode of transient global amnesia.

Not all physicians agree that transient global amnesia (TGA) is a symptom of vascular disease. However, research continues to support evidence that individuals who experience a lack of blood supply to areas responsible for memory have episodes during which memory is lost for a short period of time.

The episodes usually last minutes to hours and resolve within 24 hours. Generally, they occur only once, without returning.

There is a strong correlation between the occurrence of TGA and a history of migraine headaches. Possibly, arterial spasms that occur with migraine headaches contribute to the interruption of blood flow to the involved area.

DIFFERENTIAL DIAGNOSIS

It is essential to note that not all transient focal neurological deficits are TIAs. There are various diseases or disorders that may account for these symptoms. Brain tumors, blood glucose imbalances, seizures, arteritis (inflammation of the arteries), inner ear disease, heart problems, and deficits resulting from migraine headaches can present symptoms mimicking TIAs. Therefore it is important that a thorough history and physical examination be obtained to determine if a TIA occurred. Appropriate therapy may then be instituted.

MURMURS (BRUITS)

Along with symptoms and syndromes such as those previously mentioned, there are physical findings or signs that suggest a disturbance in blood flow. One such finding is the presence of a murmur, or bruit. A bruit is an abnormal sound noted while listening with a stethoscope to areas supplying blood. There are numerous causes that may contribute to the presence of a bruit: low red blood cell count (anemia), certain types of tumor (meningiomas, glomus tumors), shunts (artificially created passages that connect two main channels and divert blood flow from one to the other; contribute to a bruit particularly in hemodialysis patients), and arteriovenous malformations (AVMs; abnormal communications between the arterial and venous systems).

A bruit can also be present because of atherosclerosis of the arteries in the neck or heart. The presence of plaque and subsequent narrowing of an artery makes the smooth flow of blood increasingly difficult. Thus as blood attempts to flow through smaller areas, turbulence occurs and a bruit results. This disturbance is much like the sound created when water flows through a stream filled with rocks.

Some bruits occur with or without symptoms of a TIA or stroke. The bruits noted with no other symptoms that would indicate difficulty with blood flow are referred to as asymptomatic bruits. It is noted that 1 to 3% of patients per year with asymptomatic bruits can go on to have a stroke.

A higher-pitched bruit is of greater concern as it indicates advanced narrowing (stenosis) of the artery. The blood flow here produces an increased sound when it tries to pass through a small area.

The absence of a bruit does not necessarily mean that an artery is disease-free. Often the artery is narrowed to such an extent that blood flowing through it is minimal. Thus with little or no flow available, detecting a bruit is difficult.

The area in which a bruit is heard is not necessarily an indication to the location of disease. Noises may radiate from the heart through the arteries in the neck, possibly misleading one to assume there is disease in an area where it does not exist. Thus a thorough evaluation of bruits, noting their source and degree of severity, is important so as to observe signs that may signal a stroke.

The signs and symptoms of a stroke mentioned here are useful to the patient, family, and physician. Appropriate treatment must be started to prevent a stroke when warning signs are noted. If these signs persist and a stroke ensues, the symptoms indicate to the physician the type of stroke and the area of the brain that is affected. An appropriate plan of management can then be instituted.

4

Examining the Patient

Most stroke-suspected individuals are seen in the doctor's office or the emergency room. From the moment the physician sees the patient, he begins to assess his condition. Does he walk normally, swinging both arms? Does he favor one side or another while walking with a limp? Does he respond appropriately when the physician shakes his hand and says hello? How is the strength in his arm and hand? Are his words understandable? What is his facial expression? Does it reflect his mood? Is his face symmetrical? This information is used along with the results of various other tests and the history to formulate a diagnosis.

HISTORY

A carefully taken history is one of the most important aspects of diagnosing a stroke or any other related cerebrovascular disease. The history alerts the examiner as to which specific areas during the physical and neurological examinations he should give special attention. Sometimes the symptoms that appeared at the onset of the problem have resolved or progressed by the time the patient is seen by the physician. Many patients have difficulty giving a history and remembering the order of events as they occurred. In any case, the patient should be allowed to freely describe his problem in his own words. If possible, all information obtained from the patient is confirmed by the family or friends. These persons are often able to give additional information that proves useful.

33

By fully informing the patient and family, their expectations of the examination as well as their fears and concerns are allayed. This attitude affords better communication and co-operation now and at any future contact.

After hearing the presenting problem from the patient and/or family and friends, specific questions need to be answered. What was the patient doing when the problem began, and did it begin suddenly or gradually? Did the problem come and go, or did it remain? Has the condition improved or worsened? Has more than one attack occurred? If so, were they all the same?

The physician also needs to ask about any items that were not covered with the presenting problem. For instance, were there any changes in memory or personality noted? Did the patient have a headache prior to or with the problem? Was there any trauma to the head? If so, was there unconsciousness? If unconsciousness occurred, how long did it last? Was there a convulsion? Were there any problems noted with speech, reading, or writing? Did a change in vision occur? Was there any difficulty with hearing or maintaining balance? Did any weakness or numbness occur that involved any part of the body? Was there any loss of bowel or bladder function?

Determining the medications the patient has been taking, if any, and if he has actually been taking them adds essential information. Did the patient forget his high blood pressure pill or his insulin injection? Is he having a reaction that could be attributed to his medication, rather than the problem being a stroke-related disease? Was he taking anything other than prescription drugs? Does he have any allergies?

A history of past medical conditions determines if specific conditions may add to or complicate the picture. Of concern are conditions such as high blood pressure, heart attacks, diabetes, low red blood cell count (anemia), and a history of previous TIAs and/or stroke. Has the patient had a previous head injury, which would aid in determining if a chronic subdural hematoma exists?

Obtaining a history of the health of the patient's family is useful, as it may give clues to familial heart and brain diseases. As was discussed earlier, heredity does play a role in increasing one's risk for stroke.

Noting social habits such as smoking and alcohol is useful. How much does the patient smoke? How long has he done so? Is he a heavy drinker? Has he fallen and injured his head while being intoxicated?

The physician also needs to be aware of stresses the patient may have been under during work, his home life, or both. Has there been a change in his work or social activities?

GENERAL AND NEUROVASCULAR EXAMINATION

An assessment of the blood pressure and pulse is an essential part of the examination. If possible, the blood pressure is measured while the patient is both lying down and standing, and in both arms. A lower pressure on standing may alert the physician that there is insufficient blood flow in the legs and feet. Differences in the two arms may be indicative of a subclavian steal syndrome, as noted in Chapter 3.

The skin is examined for the presence of small reddened lesions indicating abnormalities in blood flow. These lesions are particularly noted along the face and conjunctiva on the eye. A reddened face may be seen with polycythemia vera, a condition discussed in Chapter 1.

Comparison of the pulses may also indicate disease of the neurovascular system. The carotid arteries are palpated gently and not at the same time, so as to avoid the risk of causing a carotid sinus reflex. The remainder of the pulses are palpated simultaneously. Any decrease or delay noted while comparing the radial pulses may be indicative of the subclavian steal syndrome. The facial and temporal arteries are supplied by the external carotid system. Decreased facial or temporal pulses are suggestive of disease of that particular artery or of the external carotid artery. Pulses increased in the external carotid distribution may be indicative of poor to no blood flow in the internal carotid arteries, as the flow increases.

As diseases of the heart and brain are frequently associated, careful attention is given to the heart. A murmur (bruit) or disturbance of blood flow may indicate hardening of the arteries. A stethoscope is used to listen to the heart and the subclavian, carotid, and ophthalmic arteries for the presence of a bruit.

A screening neurological examination is done in order to evaluate the function of the brain. Specific areas of the brain are responsible for particular actions. Therefore an inability to perform a particular act indicates malfunctioning in a particular area. A thorough evaluation is useful.

TESTING MENTAL FUNCTION

As was stated earlier, at the initial observation and during the history taking certain neurological information can be obtained. In particular, pertinent facts about the patient's mental function may be assessed quickly during this time.

The most important factor to be determined is the patient's level of consciousness. Is he alert and oriented? Or is he drowsy? Does he respond to pain? Is he in a coma and unresponsive?

Another important aspect is the overall appearance and behavior of the patient. What is his state of cleanliness and grooming? What is his attitude? Does he pay attention? Are commands followed?

The patient's intellectual function may be determined during the initial conversation as well. Is he aware of the date, place, and day of the week? Can he recall past events? Can he retain digits or names of objects given to him? The patient's ability to calculate by addition, subtraction, and multiplication is also noted. Consideration is given here to the amount of education the patient has received.

Throughout the history taking, any disorders of speech are

assessed. Does the patient have difficulty verbalizing what he wants to say? Can he understand what is being said to him? Are his words slurred? Can he interpret written language? If there are difficulties with communication, certain aspects of the examination may be more difficult to obtain. The examiner and family members must exhibit patience, thereby aiding the patient who most likely is extraordinarily stressed.

TESTING CRANIAL NERVE FUNCTION

Specific nerves connect directly with the brain and enable us to perform various functions. When a stroke occurs, some of these nerves may be affected. Thus the ability to smell, see, swallow, and hear, for instance, may be impaired. The examiner tests each of the 12 cranial nerves to determine the area the stroke has affected and the extent of damage that has occurred.

Cranial nerve I. The first cranial nerve controls the sense of smell. Each nostril is checked separately for familiar odors, such as coffee or tobacco.

Cranial nerve II. The second cranial nerve allows the patient to see. Does he wear corrective lenses? Does he have a normal field of vision? Can he see well at the periphery, or does he have a blind spot? An ophthalmoscope allows the examiner to observe the retina and blood vessels to determine if there is an abnormality.

Cranial nerves III, IV, and VI. The third, fourth, and sixth cranial nerves are tested together, as all are concerned with eye movements. A deficit here can be noted by having the patient follow the examiner's fingers in all directions of gaze. The third cranial nerve is also responsible for constriction of the pupils and elevation of the eyelids.

Cranial nerve V. The fifth cranial nerve provides sensation to the face and the ability to bite. The patient's blinking response, which is also a function of the fifth nerve, can be tested by touching a wisp of cotton to the cornea of the eye.

Cranial nerve VII. The seventh cranial nerve allows movement of the facial muscles. Is there any asymmetry when the patient smiles, wrinkles his forehead, or raises his eyebrows? There is also a sensory component to this nerve that notes the sensation of the front part of the tongue on each side. Sugar and salt are generally used to test this function.

Cranial nerve VIII. The eighth cranial nerve is concerned with the ability to hear and maintain balance. Can the patient hear a watch ticking when it is held to each ear? Does he properly identify the sound being moved away? Generally, tests that may determine problems with ringing in the ears, a spinning sensation, and/or difficulty with balance are more involved and are not done routinely. However, if the patient gives a history of such problems, appropriate tests should be performed.

Cranial nerves IX and X. The ninth and tenth cranial nerves are tested together by noting the patient's ability to swallow, the symmetrical movements of the soft palate when he is asked to say "ah," and the ability to speak clearly without hoarseness.

Cranial nerve XI. The eleventh cranial nerve controls shoulder strength. Can the patient shrug his shoulders against resistance?

Cranial nerve XII. The twelfth cranial nerve controls the strength of the tongue. Can the patient protrude his tongue and move it from side to side? Can he press his tongue against the side of his cheeks?

TESTING MOTOR AND SENSORY FUNCTION

In addition to cranial nerve testing, it is important to assess motor and sensory function. Loss of movement and sensation are common problems encountered by the stroke patient, as discussed previously.

Muscle Strength and Gait

The ability to initiate, maintain, and control movement is a function of the motor system. A comparison of the mass, tone, and strength of the muscle groups determines if there is an abnormality.

The examiner needs to determine if the muscles in the arms and legs are the same size and if there is any rigidity or spasticity present. Is there any difference in the strength? How is the grip in the hands? Can the patient squat and stand without assistance? Can he walk on his toes and heels? Does he have a normal gait? Observing the gait allows the examiner to quickly assess any weakness or lack of coordination.

Reflexes

Using a small rubber hammer, the reflexes can be examined to determine if they are normal, increased, or decreased. The end of the hammer or a key is used to test reflex responses on the bottom of the feet.

Sensation

There are specific instruments used to determine a patient's response to soft touch, pain, temperature, vibration, and position sense. Generally each side of the body is tested and compared to the other side. A wisp of cotton tests one's sensation to soft touch, whereas a sharp pin determines the response to pain. A tuning fork is useful for testing vibration sense. The use of hot and cold items evaluates the response to temperature. Other tests—such as one in which the patient stands with eyes closed, feet together, and arms extended—judge position sense.

Cerebellar Function

Tests of cerebellar function evaluate the patient's execution of coordination and fine movements. The ability to maintain balance is also controlled by the cerebellum. The physician may want to see if the patient can keep his balance while walking with one foot in front of the other, heel to toe. Can he perform rapid alternating movements, such as patting his knees with the palms and back of his hands? A familiar test noting coordination is having the patient touch his index finger to his own nose and then to the physician's finger. The physician changes the position of his finger, making the test more difficult. This procedure is done rapidly several times while testing each hand.

These tests are a few examples by which cerebellar function is observed. There are other tests in which the physician can determine if actions are performed accurately and smoothly. The inability to do so may indicate cerebellar disease.

COMATOSE PATIENTS

Some strokes cause unconsciousness. A brief history may be obtained by the family or anyone with the patient at the time. If no one is available, information on the patient such as a history of allergies, medications he is taking, or any conditions he may have as indicated by a medical alert band is pertinent.

The most important concern when examining the comatose patient is determining if he has an adequate airway (can he breathe adequately). Vital signs such as blood pressure, pulse, and temperature must be maintained within normal limits. The level of consciousness, as discussed earlier, is a major factor to observe. A response to painful stimuli while in a coma is a more positive sign than no response at all. The motor system can be assessed by noting any movement as well as any response to the stimuli. A decrease in the level of consciousness is an indication of deterioration in the patient's condition.

OTHER TESTS

Other aspects of the neurological examination, such as pupillary response and reflexes, can be assessed without patient cooperation. The remainder of the examination may be performed as the patient's condition improves.

5

Tests Used for Diagnosis and Management of Stroke

The best way to determine that a patient has had a stroke is by taking a careful history and performing a thorough examination. However, in order to identify precisely its cause and location, other tests are necessary that cannot be done at the bedside. These tests fall into two categories: (a) tests specifically designed to locate the disorder within the brain and (b) more general tests to determine the health of the patient and identify the cause of the problem (which, for example, might come from the heart or another part of the body but localize in the brain).

In this chapter we describe some of these tests so that when they are ordered those involved will know why they are done and what the results may mean. By being aware of how they are done and what they can tell us, both the patient and the family can be emotionally prepared and not frightened or anxious about them.

BLOOD TESTS

The blood that circulates through the body is a liquid that contains a large number of dissolved chemicals plus cells suspended in the fast-flowing stream. The heart propels the blood through the body, which derives its nutrition from the blood; the body's cells also eliminate their waste products (from metabolism) by excreting them into the blood; therefore, de-

42

pending on the part of the bloodstream from which the sample is taken, one finds different quantities of various chemicals. For example, the arterial side contains oxygen, which has been obtained from the lungs when the arterial blood passes through them. The arterial blood then passes through the tissues, where the oxygen is withdrawn; venous blood thus has much less oxygen in it. Venous blood, on the other hand, has more carbon dioxide than does arterial blood because carbon dioxide is formed during the metabolism of tissue and is passed into the venous circulation to be got rid of when the veins pass through the lungs. The same is true of blood glucose.

Because it is easier blood samples are usually obtained from a vein, but it is also possible to withdraw blood from an artery—and in some cases an arterial sample is essential. When blood is withdrawn from the body and allowed to sit for a few minutes, it normally forms a clot, which is rather like Jello in consistency. Such blood clots (which may also be found in the body under certain conditions) are designed to stop the bleeding after a wound has occurred. (Blood clotting is described later on.) After the blood has clotted, the serum, which is a clear fluid, is left and is the part of the blood that contains all the materials that have been dissolved, including proteins, carbohydrates, fats, and other chemicals. Contained within the blood clot itself is all the particulate matter, especially the red and white blood cells and the platelets.

These cells are manufactured in the bone marrow, which is contained in the porous bones of the body, particularly, the thoracic cage, the vertebrae, and some of the long bones. This cell-producing system is a very active one because normally red blood cells live for only about 3 months before they die, white blood cells live only a few hours, and platelets even less. Therefore the body must continually replace these cells. In normal people the system is in a perfect balance: The number of red blood cells, white blood cells, and platelets being destroyed is perfectly compensated by the number of new ones being produced and released into the system. In contrast, an infection somewhere in the body causes an outpouring of new white blood cells to combat the infection so that the white blood count becomes elevated; in other cases platelets become too many or too few for a variety of reasons. In each of these situations abnormalities in the cerebral circulation may result.

A complete blood count (CBC) indicates how many red blood cells and white blood cells are in a cubic centimeter of blood, among other measurements. Red blood cells have the important task of carrying hemoglobin. Hemoglobin gives blood a red color and is responsible for transporting oxygen from the lungs to other organs. Normal red blood cell values are for men 5.4 ± 0.7 million cells per cubic milliliter (mm^3) and for women 4.8 ± 0.6 million cells/mm^3. Low red blood count values may indicate anemia and cause a deficient supply of oxygen to the brain. Elevated values occur when there are too many cells, which causes the blood to sludge, making flow difficult.

The main function of white blood cells is to prevent or fight infection. Normal values are 4,800 to 10,800 cells/mm^3.

A platelet count may also be necessary to determine the number of platelets circulating in the blood. Normal values are 130,000 to 400,000 platelets/mm^3. Platelets circulate in the bloodstream and often stick to uneven or damaged surfaces in an effort to repair these areas. Clumping of platelets on the wall of an artery can cause immense harm because they may block the artery, thereby preventing adequate blood flow. In some situations a portion of the platelet clump breaks off and eventually lodges in an artery too small for it to pass, thereby becoming an embolism.

Testing for Inflammation

An erythrocyte sedimentation rate (ESR) may also be determined along with the CBC. An elevated ESR, or "sed rate,'' can be caused by inflammation of the arteries (arteritis) or infection. Normal values for men are 10 to 20 mm/hour; values for women are 10 to 30 mm/hour.

Testing for Fats in the Blood

There are three fats that circulate in the blood: cholesterol, triglycerides, lipoprotein. All come from the foods we eat. If we consume too great a quantity or if our metabolism is abnormal, the blood levels of various substances become elevated. In order to eliminate the effect of food intake on laboratory results, the blood must be withdrawn from the body after a 12-hour fast. Elevated amounts of cholesterol and fats contribute to hardening of the arteries (arteriosclerosis), thus making blood flow through the narrowed arteries difficult. The normal value for cholesterol is 110 to 250 mg per deciliter (dl) and for triglycerides 10 to 150 mg/dl.

Testing for Diabetes

Diabetes, discussed in Chapter 1, occurs when there is an excessive level of glucose in the blood because of the body's inability to metabolize glucose properly. Thus after a meal the blood glucose level automatically increases. It should return to normal levels within 2 hours because the liver and other tissues consume the glucose or store it. If the blood glucose content becomes excessively high, glucose may be excreted in the urine.

The controlling factor is insulin, a hormone secreted into the bloodstream by the pancreas. Insulin facilitates the transfer of glucose from blood to tissues; it also promotes storage of glucose by the liver and to a lesser degree by other organs. Without enough insulin a person develops diabetes mellitus. Not only does the blood glucose level rise, causing undesirable side effects, but tissues of the body lose their ability to metabolize it normally, creating abnormalities in their various functions.

A glucose level that is extremely high may indicate that not enough insulin is being produced. Another way to check for diabetes is to have the individual eat a large meal and have his blood level assayed 2 hours later. A level of 140 mg/dl or more is considered an indication of diabetes.

Individuals with diabetes mellitus are likely to develop damage to their arteries over a period of time. Moreover, a sudden increase or decrease in blood glucose may cause one to exhibit symptoms that are similar to those thought otherwise to be TIAs.

Thyroid Tests

The hormones secreted by the thyroid gland are essential for maintaining the body's metabolism—most importantly, metabolism in the brain. Below-normal levels cause one to become sluggish and lethargic and to think slowly. Elevated levels cause hypermetabolism, irritability, and increased appetite. Testing for levels of these hormones in the blood enables one to determine if the symptoms, which mimic those of a stroke, are actually due to decreased thyroid function.

A coagulation profile, consisting of a prothrombin time (PT) and partial thromboplastin time (PTT), is used to monitor the effectiveness of medications prescribed to thin the blood (anticoagulants). These medications also minimize the chance of blood clots that may lodge in vessels, thereby impairing blood flow and subsequently causing a stroke.

The prothrombin time works as a control for the drug warfarin (Coumadin), whereas the partial thromboplastin time is used to keep an eye on heparin levels in the blood. If the patient is taking either of these blood "thinners," a daily blood profile is done. It is necessary because the physician must be aware of any need to adjust the patient's dosage.

TESTS OF BRAIN FUNCTION

Computed Cranial Tomography

Computed cranial tomography (CCT), sometimes referred to as the CT (or CAT) scan, involves the use of a computer along with a special x-ray machine. The patient lies flat, with his head placed in a rotating machine that sends a beam of x-rays through the head. Depending on the structures it passes through, more or fewer x-rays reach the other side. Whatever does go through is recorded in a computer, and after the beam has rotated completely around the head this recording can be printed out as a picture of the brain. Sometimes an x-ray-opaque dye is injected into the vein to enhance the contrast between the brain and the blood vessels.

The complications with this procedure are minimal, the most common being an allergic reaction to the dye. Generally, a small amount of dye is injected into the vein, and if no reaction is noted the procedure continues. Forcing fluids to flush the kidneys after the dye is injected helps prevent kidney complications.

Skull X-Ray Studies

X-ray films of the head are often useful for identifying a fracture or other signs of head injury that may indicate the presence of a brain hemorrhage. Skull x-ray studies have no serious side effects and are not harmful to the patient.

Brain Scan

Brain scans use a small amount of radioactive dye and a radiation counter to show areas of the brain not seen on regular x-ray pictures. They can be helpful for differentiating certain types of stroke as well as determining if the problem is a tumor, a blood clot, or a blocked artery.

A small amount of radioactive material is injected into a vein in the arm, after which the counter is placed close to the head. Approximately 1.5 hours later the rest of the pictures are taken, this portion of the procedure lasting approximately 1 hour. If the patient is in the hospital, he may be returned to his room between the first and final picture-taking sessions. Complications from this procedure are minimal. An increased intake of fluids is encouraged to help eliminate the dye from the kidneys.

Magnetic Resonance Imaging

A new type of test that beautifully depicts the anatomy of the brain is the magnetic resonance imaging (MRI) scan. It involves the use of magnetic and low-energy radiowaves to produce a series of pictures of the head. No x-rays, dye, or radioactive materials are used as with the CT or brain scan.

In most but not all scanners, rather than only the head being placed in the scanner, as with the CT scan, the entire body is rolled into a tunnel-shaped machine. Surrounding this tunnel is a large magnet with a radio transmitter and receiver. The magnet is attracted to certain areas of the human body containing hydrogen, which is mostly in the form of water. Radio signals are then transmitted indicating this attraction, and a picture is formed.

Because metal objects may interfere with the scan, jewelry, glasses, or other materials containing metal must be removed. If the patient has had a prior surgical procedure requiring metal clips or has a cardiac pacemaker or an artificial metallic joint, the scan may be impossible to perform.

It is important for the patient to be cooperative and not move during the testing. Any movement results in blurring of the pictures. The procedure generally takes 40 to 50 minutes to perform. No harmful side effects have been noted with this scan.

The MRI scan has been shown to identify certain strokes,

tumors, or other neurological diseases possibly not seen with the CT scan.

Cerebral Angiography

The cerebral angiogram or arteriogram is useful for noting areas of blood vessel narrowing or obstruction. An x-ray-opaque dye is injected into the bloodstream while x-ray films are obtained. Usually the femoral artery, located at the groin, is the site chosen for insertion of a small tube (catheter). The dye is then injected through the catheter, and the pathway of the dye is followed to observe the vessels of the brain.

Angiography is absolutely contraindicated for patients who have experienced a recent heart attack and/or who have breathing problems. Conditions such as malignant hypertension, allergies to the contrast dye, and anticoagulant therapy are relative contraindications. Some physicians consider age to be a contraindication, but the overall physical condition of the patient at any age seems to be of more importance.

In addition to the contraindications noted, there are complications associated with this study; the mortality rate is low, however. The more commonly seen serious problems involve renal damage, bleeding from the puncture site, transient ischemic attacks (TIAs), and stroke.

Renal or kidney problems can occur when the dye is not excreted rapidly or thoroughly enough. Thus it is important to increase fluid intake after the procedure in order to prevent kidney failure.

Another complication that may occur is bleeding from the puncture site. After the test is completed and the catheter is withdrawn, pressure is applied to the site for approximately 10 minutes. This pressure keeps bleeding from occurring under the skin. Pulses are checked at the groin, leg, and foot to ensure that there is adequate blood flow throughout the artery.

A TIA or stroke may also occur during angiography, although it is unusual. The reason for this problem is that upon working the catheter through the artery a piece of plaque or a platelet clump may be loosened from the artery wall. This loosened debris can then travel throughout the bloodstream and lodge in an area too small for it to pass through, causing a TIA or stroke—which one depends on the length of time the artery is blocked. Generally, a medication such as aspirin is given to the patient to prevent such problems. (Aspirin works as an antiplatelet agent.)

Angiography has also been shown to be effective not only for diagnosing but for treating diseases. For instance, in cases of hemorrhage by injecting a form of clotting agent through a catheter and blocking the vessel bleeding can be stopped.

Passing tiny balloons through a narrowed or blocked blood vessels has also proved to be an effective method for opening or widening the area. The balloon is moved into position using the catheter as a guide and is then inflated, thereby widening and thus opening the vessel.

The benefits of angiography often outweigh the risks, as important information may be obtained with this test that has not previously been shown with others. The physician can decide along with the patient and family the relative importance of having this test performed.

Digital Subtraction Angiography

Another procedure that also detects narrowing and/or obstruction in the arteries is the digital subtraction angiogram. The procedure is similar to that described for cerebral angiography. The major difference is that the small tube (catheter) is inserted into a vein, not an artery. The location is usually in the arm. Dye is then injected into the vein and travels to the heart, where a certain amount enters the arteries. X-ray pictures are obtained after the dye is injected.

This procedure is contraindicated if the patient is allergic to the contrast dye. The most common complication is renal or kidney problems, described earlier for cerebral angiography.

As this test is relatively new, there remains a question as to how successful it is at determining blockage of the arteries. The procedure appears less likely to cause a stroke or a TIA, and so much effort will be put into making it a more effective study.

Ultrasound Procedures

Doppler Scans and B-Scans

Ultrasound has become an effective method for detecting narrowing (stenosis) of the arteries. As the sound beams penetrate a moving target, such as blood, a reflection is given that indicates any areas of stenosis.

The carotid doppler scan is concerned with noting the flow of blood through the carotid arteries (Fig. 4). By placing the instrument probe at the location of the carotid arteries on the neck, one can note flow through the common, external, and internal carotid arteries. Also, the flow through the ophthalmic artery can be observed by placing the probe over the patient's closed eye. This technique is particularly useful in patients who are experiencing temporary blindness in an eye (amaurosis fugax), as the difficulty with blood flow can be observed.

The B-mode (brightness mode), or real-time, scan notes the width of the artery and looks for atherosclerotic thickening. The latter is indicated by reflected or brightened areas on the scan. The images shown on the scan are produced rapidly under the conditions (real time) it actually occurs (Fig. 5).

Echocardiogram

The echocardiogram also involves the use of ultrasound waves necessary for imaging the heart. An instrument emitting

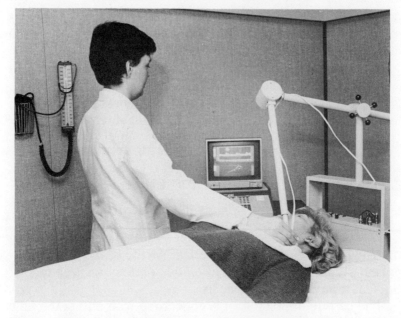

FIG. 4.   The carotid doppler scan notes the flow of blood through the carotid arteries via the use of ultrasound beams.

sound waves is placed over the heart, and the picture recorded from these sound waves enables one to observe for emboli or any cardiac abnormalities that may contribute to stroke.

Amplifying Stethoscope

Carotid phonoangiography (CPA) is another technique used in the ultrasound laboratory for the purpose of detecting bruits (murmurs). An instrument similar to a stethoscope, but which contains a microphone used for amplification of sound, is placed on the carotid artery at three locations: at the base of the neck, the middle of the neck [the area where the common carotid artery divides into the internal and external carotid arteries (bifurcation)], and the top of the jaw (mandible).

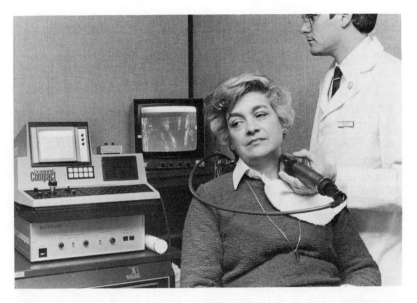

FIG. 5. Real time of B-mode scanning indicates if there is atherosclerotic thickening present on the artery walls.

If a bruit is heard, it is essential for the observer to note the location, duration, pitch, and quality. This test is often helpful for locating the origin of a bruit because with the aid of amplification one can note whether the bruit is referred from the heart or originates in the carotid artery itself. Such a distinction may prove too difficult with an ordinary stethoscope.

Oculoplethysmography

Oculoplethysmography (OPG) is sometimes used in the ultrasound laboratory as an additional test to evaluate disease from the arteries in the neck to the eyes. Remember, the first major branch of the internal carotid artery is the ophthalmic artery, which supplies the eyes. The ophthalmic artery is therefore accessible to evaluation by this procedure; that is, blood flow to the eyes is monitored.

There are two possible techniques used for this test. The selection of one or the other technique depends on the equipment available and the physician's preference. Both tests supply the same information.

There are no specific preparations required for OPG testing. Clips are placed on the ears and cups on the eyes during the test. Earlobe massage and eyedrops containing a numbing agent aid in making the equipment used more tolerable. Recordings of pulsations or pressure in the eyes are taken as an indicator of internal carotid artery flow. These recordings are compared to pulsations obtained from the earlobes, which indicate external carotid flow. Any difference noted between the pulsations may indicate blockage of one of the arteries.

There are specific considerations to note before performing the test. The patient must be aware that cooperation is essential, as eye movement may result in false recordings. Dimming, loss of vision, or both may occur for 5 to 10 seconds when pressure is applied to compress the artery in the eye using one of the techniques.

An allergy to plastic or local anesthetics, a history of retinal detachment, eye injury or eye surgery within the past 6 months, and/or a prosthetic eye are contraindications. A patient with a history of glaucoma may have the test performed, although one should be aware that inaccurate readings may result.

The actual testing time is approximately 30 minutes. The patient must be reminded that the eyes remain numb for 15 to 20 minutes after testing. Caution is taken to avoid rubbing the eyes and to prevent foreign objects from being introduced.

Comment

The ultrasound tests described above are generally without risk. Better results are usually obtained if the patient is cooperative, as movement of the patient makes scanning more difficult.

Regional Cerebral Blood Flow

The regional cerebral blood flow (rCBF) study has become important in localizing areas of the brain affected by stroke. Patients inhale an inert gas, xenon, a radioactive isotope, which subsequently is traced through the brain, indicating locations not receiving sufficient blood. The gas is harmless and causes no harmful effects. In fact, it is no more harmful than a single chest x-ray.

Electroencephalogram

The electroencephalogram (EEG) monitors the electrical activity of the brain. By placing electrodes on the scalp this activity can be recorded, much as the electrocardiogram (ECG) is used to monitor the heart rate.

The EEG is most commonly obtained to diagnose seizures or tumors, although it can be useful for evaluating a patient who has had a stroke. Often similar symptoms occur with these disorders, and it is important to be aware of the accurate diagnosis. Seizures may occur after a stroke because of the irritation of brain tissue that results from interruption of the blood supply.

Sometimes the patient is sleep deprived or sedated for this test. Either of these situations may induce a seizure that would not be noted under other conditions. These situations may make the brain more susceptible to a seizure. Therefore, the physician can determine the type of seizure and manage it appropriately.

Lumbar Puncture

A lumbar puncture, or spinal tap, is performed on some patients as an aid in determining the proper treatment. A needle is placed into the spinal canal through the patient's back in order to obtain a small amount of cerebrospinal fluid (CSF) and to measure the pressure inside the central nervous system (CNS). The test is particularly useful when medication to thin the blood (anticoagulant) is being considered; in such cases it is important to know if there has been bleeding into the brain. If such bleeding has occurred, another type of medication may be needed.

The most common complication of this test is a headache. Forcing fluids and remaining flat in bed for approximately 8 hours after the test help prevent this side effect. The time required in bed varies, of course, according to the patient's condition and the physician's judgment.

Comment

Some of the tests discussed above are done only during the patient's hospitalization. Others may be repeated in order to more effectively manage treatment and follow-up. Specific tests may not be performed on all patients, as the physician may not consider them necessary. Remember that discussions with the medical staff serve to inform both patient and family of the specific plan chosen for the individual patient.

6

Management of Stroke

In other chapters the means by which strokes can often be prevented—by reducing risk factors—were discussed. Also emphasized was the idea that prevention is far better than treatment. In this chapter the means by which stroke can be prevented in patients who have warning symptoms (transient ischemic attacks) are discussed, as are the ways to limit damage to the brain in people who are already suffering with an advancing stroke.

TRANSIENT ISCHEMIC ATTACKS

Transient ischemic attacks (TIAs)—warning signals that a full-blown stroke may take place—are usually caused by small emboli that progress through the bloodstream to lodge in smaller vessels within the brain, causing temporary loss of blood flow. Most cerebral infarctions result from large blood clots that obstruct a blood vessel permanently. The mechanisms of TIAs and stroke are thus the same. Although the figures vary among reports, about one-third of patients who eventually have cerebral infarctions have warnings via TIAs before the stroke occurs. Some TIAs occur in the eye, where they cause temporary blindness or blind spots; others occur in either the right or left cerebral hemisphere, causing symptoms of deficits, as described in Chapter 3.

When TIAs occur they constitute an emergency situation until the doctor has found out why they are occurring and, when possible, removes the cause. Because there are many causes, treatments vary. For example, in some cases the blood is too thick because of too many red blood cells or platelets, and the treatment is designed to correct this abnormality. In other cases the TIA results from emboli from the heart due to abnormal rhythms, which should be corrected. In most cases, however, TIAs are due to atherosclerotic plaques located in the artery of the neck (carotid artery); when the disease becomes sufficiently advanced, a blood clot forms on the inner surface of the artery. This clot, for one reason or another, may fragment, and the fragments go to the distant arteries and lodge there.

Because a plaque in the carotid artery is usually located where it can be removed many physicians advocate surgery (endarterectomy). Others, pointing to the statistics in the literature, say that the efficacy of surgery has not been proved beyond a shadow of a doubt, that the risk of complications (which might even include death) runs anywhere from 3 to 15%, and that it is likely that the patient will eventually die with a heart attack anyway, so why perform surgery? Instead, they advocate the use of platelet antiaggregants or anticoagulant drugs as well as reduction of risk factors.

These two forms of management each have their strong proponents. We recommend an intermediate position and suggest that both forms of management be considered for different categories of patients. We believe that people who are in excellent health, whose bodies are "physiologically young," and who have a long life expectancy should be strongly considered for having a carotid endarterectomy if a single plaque of atherosclerosis is found at the carotid bifurcation, particularly if this plaque is almost blocking the artery and if it has caused TIAs. Although there is no hard evidence to prove it, logic suggests that such advanced disease would have little likelihood of healing spontaneously and that it had best be removed before it produces a devastating stroke.

On the other hand, if the patient is elderly or has many other diseases and a short life expectancy, treatment is best done medically, because not only is there the risk of surgery but the likelihood of dying of some intercurrent disease is excessive. It is therefore not worthwhile for the patient to undertake an immediate risk for what would be unlikely long-term gain.

Whenever surgical management is chosen, one must be aware that the treatment is designed only to remove a life-threatening patch of disease in 1 or 2 inches of artery when in fact the lesions (atherosclerotic plaques) are probably located here and there throughout the entire arterial system. Because of this disseminated disease, in addition to surgery all patients must have medical management, particularly to reduce any risk factors that may be present.

Few doctors recommend surgery for disease of the vertebrobasilar arterial system because the arteries are tightly encased in the bone of the cervical spine. For this group of patients, management by medical means, including platelet antiaggregants and blood pressure control, seems best. In some instances the disease of these posterior circulation arteries is precipitated by a change of head position, whereas in others trauma to the vertebrae in the neck is the cause, as with "whiplash" injuries. In such cases the artery is pinched by movement of the bone, and at least in some cases further damage can be prevented by controlling the head and neck movements.

There has been great interest in bypass operations, which allow blood to move around obstructions. Although this method has been successful in the coronary artery (the circulation of the heart), it has not proved useful for the cerebral circulation, at least according to the data published on the randomized prospective trial of extracranial to intracranial bypass in patients who have had TIAs and cerebral infarction. Although these results have been challenged, the weight of evidence is that such operations should seldom be performed and then only in unusual circumstances in institutions where special facilities are available and the surgeons are particularly skillful. Who, if anyone, needs this type of surgery is a medical judgment. Surgeons are able to perform the procedure, but the *need* for the surgery is still debated.

REVERSIBLE ISCHEMIC NEUROLOGICAL DEFICIT

The management of patients with the more prolonged neurological deficits is more problematical than that of patients with TIAs. By definition, a patient who has a TIA is normal before 24 hours has elapsed. The patient with reversible ischemic neurological deficit (RIND) might have neurological deficit for as long as a week, but does not have evidence of infarction on computed tomography (CT) scan or magnetic resonance imaging (MRI). In such cases of carotid artery occlusion (blockage) that has caused continued deficit without change in the brain, some physicians advocate emergency arteriography and endarterectomy to restore the circulation. Therefore it is advisable to have an emergency evaluation of the patient, including noninvasive studies and perhaps arteriography, to determine if the artery is fully closed. In patients with tight stenosis or occlusion, reconstructive surgery may be useful.

Often the doctor uses anticoagulants, particularly heparin or warfarin, to thin the blood and make it less coagulable so that further blood clots do not accumulate during the time the patient's brain has poor circulation. When the flow of blood slows and the pressure is reduced distal to an occlusion (obstruction), stagnation of the flow often results in clotting. Under these circumstances, the anticoagulant is extremely useful.

Other physicians suggest reducing the number of coagulable elements within the blood by removing a pint of blood (sometimes even more) to make the blood thinner (less viscous). Surprisingly, the use of oxygen or vasodilators to open the blood vessels and nerve blocks is ineffective and does not increase the patient's margin of recovery.

ESTABLISHED INFARCTION

When brain tissue loses its blood supply it dies quickly, resulting in an infarction. Because the tissue does not regrow, the infarction results in a permanent abnormality, or loss of function. The goal of management is to reduce or minimize this loss by keeping the marginal tissues that immediately surround the infarcted area alive so that they can recover function.

The fact that brain tissue dies quickly and does not recover does not mean that the patient cannot have function restored by substitution of other parts of the brain and other skills for the ones that have been lost. Interesting and remarkable examples of recovery do occur despite the presence of large infarctions in what would usually be considered vital parts of the brain. Recovery is particularly evident in young patients. The younger the person, the more the nervous system is plastic and can be molded and shaped to substitute one area of brain for another; as one ages this plasticity becomes less. The patient should begin to use his affected body parts as soon as possible and to keep his normal limbs exercised and ready for use. This subject is discussed in detail in Chapter 9.

One would think that oxygen and medicines that dilate the blood vessels would have a good effect in reducing the ravages of stroke. Surprisingly, exactly the opposite is true. The reason is that oxygen constricts the blood vessels that go to the brain; what is necessary, then, is to somehow accomplish the widest dilation of collateral vessels so they can carry blood to the ischemic area. This phenomenon does in fact occur as part of the infarction process. When an infarction begins, the ischemic (oxygen-deprived) tissue sends messages that cause blood vessels in the surrounding areas to dilate, if they can do so. As a consequence, the maximum amount of blood is now passing through to the brain; therefore when extra oxygen is given, it reduces the amount of blood available to the brain by constricting these collateral vessels. The use of vasodilators to open blood vessels also has a countereffect because it opens the blood vessels in the surrounding, healthy tissues even wider; the blood vessels in the damaged tissue, in contrast, are already maximally opened and cannot increase their diameters; this situation, then, causes blood to move from the damaged tissue into the more normal tissue.

There is much interest in what is called the ischemic penumbra, which is the area of reduced oxygen and glucose supply immediately surrounding the ischemic tissue. It is conceivable that in this area continued function hangs in the balance and that some increase in availability of nutrients could preserve function. There are those who believe that reducing the metabolic need of the tissue by sedation and absolute rest of the tissue is the most productive method of therapy. By doing so, it is claimed, there is considerable potential for improvement, if not full recovery, in the area surrounding the infarcted brain.

One of the major problems of patients with stroke includes the complications of bed rest. Such patients are necessarily inactive and often cannot complain or make their needs known; as a consequence, vital necessities are sometimes ignored or misinterpreted. (a) The most important rule here is to keep an adequate oxygen supply by making sure that the breathing passages remain open. All too often patients have their necks flexed or they accumulate secretions that partially obstruct their breathing. (b) Another requirement is to keep the blood pressure within normal boundaries if possible and to give the patient an adequate supply of glucose so that the brain can continue normal metabolism. If seizures are a problem, they must be stopped; one method is to use anticonvulsants in adequate dosages. (c) A third need is to provide adequate fluid intake to ensure adequate blood volume.

Other complications of bed rest begin to occur after the second or third day. Pneumonia may appear because the patient does not breathe adequately and secretions, food, or other materials are aspirated into the breathing passages.

Fluids in adequate volume are given intravenously if the patient cannot swallow, and paying careful attention to the intake of liquids and output of urine is vital. Sometime after the first week clotting in the leg veins may occur, resulting ultimately in a pulmonary embolism. Therefore movement of the legs must begin at once, and in many cases an anticoagulant is given to prevent the blood from clotting.

If the brain is swollen, some doctors believe that its reduction is important and prescribe steroids, mannitol, or glycerol. In other instances, diuretic therapy is used.

For patients with acute, evolving cerebral infarctions, anticoagulants may be necessary. On the horizon is the potential for thrombolysis (a method to dissolve the blood clot that is causing the problem). This method is currently too new to be recommended, however.

CEREBRAL HEMORRHAGE

The treatment of cerebral hemorrhage is generally similar to treatment of an acute cerebral infarction. However, here, there is the additional problem of blood escaping into the brain. Most of these patients have high blood pressure, and in these instances it is vital to reduce the blood pressure toward normal in order to help stop the flow of blood.

Depending on where the hemorrhage is located, some physicians advocate removing the blood clot, as the clot may produce pressure on adjacent, normal tissue and cause side effects—not from the bleeding but from the actual mass of the clot. There is much evidence that if the blood clot is located in appropriate areas it may be removed surgically with dramatic improvement in the patient.

In other cases the hemorrhage bleeds into the ventricles of the brain and plugs them, causing pressure to build because the flow of cerebrospinal fluid is blocked. In these cases a drain can be inserted to remove CSF or blood.

In either case, however, expert advice is necessary, and in

practice few patients actually come to surgery. In most patients with cerebral hemorrhage, strict bed rest, no visitors, and deep sedation (in the hope that the hemorrhage will stop) is the treatment of choice.

Complications of bed rest are prevented in precisely the same way as for cerebral infarction with one exception. Whereas the patient who has an infarction is moved, allowed to sit up, and possibly ambulated within days of the event, the patient with cerebral hemorrhage is kept at strict bed rest for times varying from 2 weeks to 1 month.

Patients who have subarachnoid hemorrhage are subjected to yet another form of management. In these cases the patient often has an aneurysm that becomes a neurosurgical emergency. Aneurysms, if seen on arteriogram and in approachable locations, can be clipped so they no longer represent the threat of rebleeding. Of all forms of hemorrhage, subarachnoid hemorrhage due to aneurysm is the most lethal. Therefore whenever possible the aneurysm is obliterated surgically.

CONCLUSION

The person who has an acute stroke is very seriously ill. As many as 40% of stroke victims die during the 3 months following the onset of acute stroke. There is no such thing as a truly minor stroke because the patient who has had this "minor stroke" is not only at high risk from that stroke but also has a predilection for suffering more strokes later on. As a consequence, strong measures to reduce the risk are vital. Furthermore, because not only is the patient at high risk but there is a strong suspicion that other family members may have a propensity to stroke, it is wise at the time of the stroke to counsel other blood relatives. They are told about methods they can use to reduce their potential for having a stroke themselves: Initiating good health habits and reducing risk factors are good rules.

7

Road to Recovery: Dealing with Common Stroke Problems

Once a stroke has occurred, the patient and his family are usually confronted with drastic changes in life style. The patient may be unable to speak, move, or see as he once did. His bladder and bowel functions are sometimes affected. Memory in the patient and emotional changes in both patient and family are also familiar problems. In addition to these physical, mental, and behavioral changes, alterations in work duties and finances are frequently seen.

Disabilities that result from stroke do not necessarily resolve within a specified time. It is difficult to predict what function will return and how long it will take to do so. Yet with the use of planned therapy, started as soon as the patient is able to tolerate it, many become functioning members of the family, and some can even go back to work.

The goal of rehabilitation is to enable the patient to regain as much function as possible by teaching him ways to cope with the disability or to circumvent it altogether. As many as 20 to 50% of all hospitalized stroke patients die of their initial stroke. However, of the survivors, many live more than 11 years after their attack, so that rehabilitation is important and makes it possible for some of these individuals to resume working. In some situations, rehabilitation enables patients to be more capable of caring for themselves and enables the family to keep them at home while the family members maintain their jobs. A family can save thousands of dollars a year through rehabilitation by reducing the need for specialized centers and skilled personnel.

Chapters 8 through 14 deal with common problems experienced by many stroke patients and their families. Each author chosen to address a specific problem is an expert or has had experience dealing with the specified area. They have written in such a manner that families can understand the problem and gain useful information about what they can do to help with the healing process.

8

Adjustment Problems

Steven S. Pierson

Emotions, intellect, and behavior are products of brain activity, and any of these aspects of personality can be affected by stroke. Intellectual changes can result from injury to the brain such as that which stroke causes. This change must be distinguished from response, which is an individual's attempt to adjust to other kinds of illness. As is discussed later, a loss of mental abilities can occur as a reaction to emotional upset, most commonly depression, and reverses itself once the emotional disturbance is treated. Intellectual deterioration results in a variety of manifestations and, depending on severity, greatly influences whether the person is able to resume his former responsibilities and life style.

INTELLECTUAL CHANGES

Intellectual changes following stroke vary considerably from person to person and depend on the state of the patient before the stroke, the location of the stroke, the person's previous life style, and the family structure. Each hemisphere has specific anatomical regions that control intellectual and motor functions, as discussed in previous chapters. In right-handed individuals the left hemisphere functions for language and the right hemisphere for visual-perceptual performance. In left-handed individuals the language center may be distributed in both hemispheres. Individuals vary in their "circuitry," and only general predictions can be made for the person based on the anatomical location of the stroke.

In general, right-sided brain damage results in a paralyzed left side, spatial-perceptual deficits, and a quick, impulsive behavioral style along with memory deficits in performance. With left-sided brain damage, right-sided paralysis results along with speech and language deficits, a slow, cautious behavior style, and memory deficits in language. With bilateral damage, some of each of these problems are seen.

With each of these broad categories special attention must be given to the patient's needs during the rehabilitative process. To say one type of stroke is more disabling than another is misleading. With right hemisphere damage language is usually preserved, and the person, superficially at least, appears to be less impaired; however, he may be far more functionally impaired than the patient with left hemisphere damage.

EMOTIONAL REPERCUSSIONS

When there is a breakdown in functioning due to a physical illness, repercussions are experienced in other areas of the body, most notably in one's emotional behavior. Damage to the brain (whether by external or internal means) results in alterations of emotions, thinking, personality, and behavior. Some of the emotional reactions occur as a part of a pattern and can be characterized as a normal psychological response to a personal loss.

Grief

Parallels can be drawn between what a stroke patient experiences after losing the use of part of his body and reactions that one goes through after the death of a loved one—a grief reaction. In the case of the stroke experience, this grief reaction is played out during the rehabilitation process.

Throughout the rehabilitation process the person becomes more aware of his deficits (for instance, an arm or leg that does not work), and these deficits become a major source of frustration; disappointment, anger, and other unpleasant emotions emerge and lead to further suffering. Added to this reaction are possible side effects from medications that cause emotional distress. It is perhaps best to see the grief reaction as a process characterized by three stages: protest and denial, despair and disorganization, and reorganization.

Fear

The family's reaction in many ways mirrors that of the patient, beginning with fear and ending with the reestablishment of "normality." During the first phase the status quo is disrupted by the stroke, initiating fear. Associated symptoms include confusion and emotional numbness or shock. Fear often evolves into anxiety, which is fear without a definite object or reality in sight—although the fear of having another stroke is often a real one. The response branches here to either flight or fight, two of the oldest means of reacting to perceived danger known to man. Flight is sometimes a more effective coping mechanism for reducing the likelihood of becoming bogged down in a vicious cycle of anger (i.e., toward professional caretakers, nurses, and physicians) and which commonly results in alienation, powerlessness, and subsequently more anger and fear. The underpinning of anger is fear, which is to say that fear is the primary emotion that may erupt into anger, the secondary emotion, or some of its close relatives: frustration and irritability. Ways to avoid this cycle include having one spokesperson of the stroke team deal with the family and, in turn, limit the number of family members involved with the staff; providing consistent factual and up-to-date information to the family interrupts this cycle as well.

Denial

It is unusual for the family in the flight response to actually abandon the patient; a more common response is denial. Here the family usually underestimates the degree of stroke impairment. A helpful form of intervention from the professional staff is the support of the family, helping them to function within the emotional and physical limitations they presently find themselves unable to adjust to. With the passage of time, the family and patient acknowledge the full impact of what has happened, after which the next phase—bargaining—occurs. This phase implies that there are idealistic expectations of a return to the patient's health as it once was. The staff is usually pleased with this phase as the family seems to have an unspoken consensus concerning what they will do in order to help the patient recover. This phase also runs its course as the shock wears off and the reality of the stroke limitations sets in. Depression, as inwardly directed or "impotent" anger, then manifests. This subject is discussed in detail later in the chapter.

Mourning

Mourning, though similar in presentation to depression, is according to Dr. Grady Bray in his book, *A Stroke Family Guide and Resource,* a "time of quiet release, of identifying specific losses and of emotionally letting go of unrealistic hopes, dreams and expectations." Finally, a reunion of oneself is reached in which new structure, new roles of family members, and new goals are discovered. About 20% of stroke patients adapt in fewer than 6 months, but 36% have not adapted by 2 to 3 years.

During this process one needs to give up negative emotions and develop awareness and positive attributes. The grief reaction includes a great deal of anticipation. The fear of the future, of having another stroke, is all too real. However, if the family of a stroke patient and the person himself know that these emotional reactions are phases that one can expect to go through, and that "this too shall pass," they can make some sense of this sometimes bewildering array of emotions. Although some of these emotional reactions do not seem appropriate, the more expected, "normal" or exaggerated psychological reactions can be distinguished from the psychopathological responses, which can be thought of as emotions out of control and arising without apparent cause.

Physical Illness versus Brain Damage

How much of the reaction is due to physical illness and how much is a direct result of brain damage is difficult to determine. When the frontal region of the brain, which assigns priorities to messages, is detached from the more primitive limbic system, the limbic system fires its messages uninhibited and behavior becomes erratic and unpredictable. This erratic firing releases the emotions of the animal living in the human body. The frontal region gives insight and creativity, but our humanness is given vitality by the limbic part of the brain. This linking of emotions to the brain has best been studied for the emotion anxiety, where its chemistry and geography have been traced to some degree.

Response to Stress

In modern society stress is a pervading fact of life, and there is probably no greater stress than that of a major physical illness such as stroke. The limbic system directly receives the messages of the external environment, as well as the body's internal environment, thereby setting off the "stress response." These messages from the limbic system overwhelm the frontal cortex, throwing the normally controlled emotional behavior into disequilibrium. This phenomenon is especially noticeable in those who have experienced right hemispheric strokes. In this situation "emotional incontinence" and a quick, impulsive behavioral style frequently result because of the release of uninhibited messages from the limbic system. With the insult to the brain that occurs with a stroke, rapid changes in feelings result, such as quick laughter that dies down rapidly followed by crying, sometimes without apparent cause. When asked what he really feels, the patient has a great deal of trouble getting in touch with his feelings: These emotions simply spill out.

Depression

Despite the known relations between emotional impairment and brain injury, one emotion especially—depression—in the stroke patient is generally thought to be secondary to loss or impairment of bodily functions. Although a consensus has not been reached, investigators have reported that stroke victims experience greater depression than other physically impaired (orthopedic) patients, despite the fact that they have similar physical disabilities. On the other hand, another medical scientist who studied stroke patients and those disabled from spinal cord and orthopedic injuries found that 5 years after injury there were no significant differences in the severity of depression, but both groups had increased levels of depression. Another researcher in the field found that depression increased during the first 2 years following stroke, remained relatively stable for 2 to 10 years after the stroke, and then increased again after 10 years. Thus it may be that after 5 years depression is approximately the same in physically disabled persons including those with stroke but just after or during the early period of injury there is a significant difference in the frequency of depression in the various groups. It may be that the difference is accounted for by the changes the brain has undergone during the stroke but which it then recovers as time goes on.

In a series of 103 unselected stroke outpatients, one-third

were depressed at the time of the initial interview, and two-thirds of those remained depressed for 8 to 9 months. By 1 year after the initial evaluation none of the patients were depressed. Depression after stroke, to be medically important enough to diagnose and treat, must occur in a significant number of patients and last for a long time. It must also significantly interfere with an individual's social and occupational function. Transient depression, lasting only a few days and reflecting the course of the stroke, indicates a more reactive relation. Maximum rehabilitation is usually attained by 6 months, and so depression should have cleared by this time if it were truly a reflection of a psychological reaction to physical illness (stroke). Depression continuing beyond this time indicates that there are definite biological components to the depressive events. Despite the controversy, after-stroke depression does parallel the pattern of functional depression recognized by those in the mental health field. Treatment of post-stroke depression has not been given much attention, and this area remains one of the great unmet needs of the stroke patient.

Investigators of depression in the stroke patient are finding that there are areas of the brain associated with "major" and "minor" types of depression. These two depression types may differ in severity and duration, but generally their patterns are similar. The noted exception to this statement is that major depression appears to be associated with a dementia-like or "pseudodementia" process, whereas the minor depression variety is not. Pseudodementia must in turn be distinguished from a dementing process similar to what used to be called senile dementia and now is called Alzheimer's disease. Symptoms usually associated with depression* include:

1. Depressed mood characterized by reports of feeling sad, low, blue, hopeless, despondent, gloomy, and so on

---

* This list is used with the permission of Nancy Gaby, M.D.

2. Inability to experience pleasure
3. Change in appetite, usually with weight loss
4. Sleep disturbance, usually insomnia
5. Loss of energy, fatigue, or lethargy
6. Agitation
7. Retardation or slowing of speech, thought, and movement
8. Decrease in sexual interest and activity
9. Loss of interest in work and usual activities
10. Feelings of worthlessness, self-reproach, guilt, and shame
11. Diminished ability to think or concentrate, with complaints of slowed thinking or mixed-up thoughts
12. Lowered self-esteem
13. Feelings of helplessness
14. Pessimism and hopelessness
15. Thoughts of death or suicide attempts
16. Anxiety
17. Bodily complaints

A mnemonic that some find useful for organizing these characteristics of depression is SAMPLE-IDS (p. 199, ref. 7). Id was a term of Sigmund Freud's that represented one of the psychological categories of the mind. S is for sleep, A for appetite, M for motor activity or mood, P for pleasure, L for libido (sex drive), E for energy, I for indecisiveness, D for thoughts of death, and S for shame. If four or more are positive with this mnemonic, depression is likely.

Although studies are still preliminary, it appears that the sites of damage that produce major and minor depression are also different. Here a great amount of scientific investigation and interest has taken place along with speculation about a cause. Major depression is associated with frontal left brain injury, whereas minor depression is associated with posterior lesions of either the right or the left hemisphere.

Another mood disorder associated with stroke is an indifferent, apathetic mental state with inappropriate cheerfulness. This cheerfulness is not associated with euphoria. Patients report anxiety, slowness, loss of interest, and worrying as well. This emotional pattern is recognized in those with right anterior lesions of the brain. One criticism of these studies is that those with right hemispheric lesions may not recognize depression in themselves. Some researchers believe that there is an emotional–anatomical correlation in the right hemisphere that parallels the organization for language, which is organized in the left hemisphere of right-handed individuals. Disorders of "affective" (emotional) language may lead patients not to recognize depression or to deny depression; this denial may contribute to the failure of some studies to find depression with right anterior hemispheric lesions. However, these patients also deny nonemotional symptoms such as impairment of sleep, appetite, and libido (sex drive); therefore this criticism is probably not justified.

Other factors that must be taken into consideration include intellectual impairment, activities of daily living, social functioning, and age. When comparing these factors to the severity of the depression, the significance of the stroke lesions' location to the left frontal area had the most predictive value.

Two factors cause post-stroke depression: (a) The area of brain that is injured (biological effects) is the part that controls emotion; and (b) the ability to function normally is lost, making a person no longer capable of an independent life style. One promising theory holds that in the case of biological depression changes in the chemicals that transmit nerve impulses and that have been injured by stroke discontinue producing these chemicals (neurotransmitters) in order to produce the building material (protein) for regeneration of the damaged nerve cells. Thus with reduced transmitter release comes the behavioral outcome of depression, or undue cheerfulness and apathy. These nerve cells (neurons) arise in the base of the brain near the emotional part of the brain and project into the frontal cortex and from there to the other layers in the cortex. A depressive disorder that occurs with left frontal brain injury or the undue cheerfulness and indifference with right frontal brain injury may be the outcome of a differential chemical response to injury depending on the injured part of the brain. This theory of reduced neurotransmitters is currently applied to functional depression, the most common form of emotional illness in the general population. It seems reasonable to apply this theory to stroke patients, as the production of neurotransmitters would be disrupted in stroke-damaged brain tissue.

One-fourth of the brain (frontal cortex) is unique to the human species and is a major site of mental disease. Logical, illogical, and higher cognitive functioning occur here to help moderate the limbic system input. All behavior is chemically mediated, but the question remains: Can doctors use drugs to restore a person to normal? The reactive nature of the person's response must be kept in mind, and medication should be prescribed only after careful psychiatric evaluation and interdisciplinary consultation. Of course, the effects of stroke are superimposed on the person's personality. When personality traits are at the root of a seemingly out-of-control emotional response, it is tempting to go for a "silver bullet" to absolve one of personal responsibility for those feelings.

Most stroke patients with depression do not receive medication or therapy for their depression. For those who do, the antidepressant nortriptyline seems to be effective. The elderly, who normally have frequent medical problems, should be treated cautiously. Certain stroke patients, because of other concurrent medical conditions, are not good candidates for this medication.

In summary, for the first year after stroke, findings indicate that depression is present in 30% of all stroke patients. Of those, not all had depression to the degree that it could be called a clinical illness, thereby meriting a diagnosis and specific medical intervention. Of those who were depressed 3 weeks after stroke, one-half of the surviving patients remained depressed at the end of a year. Depression seems to have a weaker-than-expected association with disability but appears to be correlated with the level of social activity, a low intelligence quotient (IQ), being a woman, living with others, and age. The reasons for the above associations are not clear. Not surprising, only 10% of depressed patients were receiving antidepressant medication. Other observations by researchers were that one-fourth of stroke patients maintained or increased social activities, though women showed more loss of social involvement than men, and 10% of caregivers had measurable stress at 6 months.

What else does it take to come back from a stroke? When one faces a whole life turnaround, how are the problems handled during the recovery phase and for the years to come? How does the family respond in a helping way to the sometimes rapid changes in emotions that arise in their loved ones? Medication cannot always treat the emotional display, so other ways of dealing with it must be found. Sometimes it depends on the family member's mood. Their threshold for toleration of seemingly irrational emotions from the stroke patient varies. Sometimes it is all right, and at other times they have to walk out of the room. Those of us who have not been stroke patients cannot imagine what it is like to be in a public place and suddenly burst out crying for no apparent reason. It is embarrassing; the person wants to stop but often cannot. It sometimes helps to start talking about something else, some other topic of conversation: the weather outside, baseball, the first thing that pops into one's mind. By doing so, you are telling the stroke patient it is all right to have emotional changes; reassurance is comforting.

Often a stroke patient talks about what he can no longer do, and it is tempting for those caring for him to focus on what he can do in an effort to discourage the person from remaining in the patient "role." It may also be an expression of the family's own denial about their loved one's illness. On the other hand, the stroke patient may simply be acknowledging his limitation. His reaction of acceptance and awareness of his condition may be out of "sync" with the attitude of the family. Thus it is important to be encouraging while recognizing the person's limitation—a fine line to walk.

Sometimes logical discussion about a problem gets through to the stroke patient, and at other times it does not. One may have a perfectly logical talk with the stroke patient, and 15 minutes later it seems as if the conversation never occurred. Communication can be straightforward at times, but with its memory function damaged by stroke the rest of the brain is just not able to work new information the way it did before. Hence the patient not only has memory problems but also language and reasoning difficulties. This person is less able to cope with problems of everyday life and is somewhat unpredictable in terms of receiving messages and responding appropriately. Some exhibit the "sundowner" syndrome in which mental fatigue causes great problems at night. Rationality may give way at this time but be restored after a good night's sleep.

Frustration and Anger

Another problem is frustration and anger. When we hurt it is acceptable to complain, but society imposes limits on how anger can be shown. This emotion in one we are taught to hold in and not to express.

A 42-year-old woman who had been the head of a company became aphasic as a result of a stroke. She felt much anger about this problem but was not able to express it openly because she, like most women in our culture, was taught early that she should not be angry. The way she dealt with it was by having her family cater to her. She was demanding, and they took on her anger passively. They tried to meet all of her demands and felt guilt almost to the point that they should have been the ones to have had the stroke. The family ended up supporting the sick role. The patient in turn became dependent on the family members, and a vicious cycle was set up.

Thus it can be seen that the family can become frustrated and experience a great deal of anger themselves. They become angry about having to focus on caring for the stroke patient as well as keeping up their own lives. The important message is not to let these feelings, especially anger, build. Anger in many ways is tied to guilt. One woman said of her situation: "When I have to leave my mother at the nursing home it makes me feel real bad . . . guilty, but I also have feelings of anger or hostility that I cannot shake." Another woman finally said to her husband: "I didn't have the stroke, you did. I'm sorry, and I'll help you as best I can, but you're going to have to help yourself and me." In each case issues were left to build, and both anger and guilt played parts. In the latter case the patient's wife felt much relieved—she had been able to "let go."

A helpful way of handling emotional conflict is with group activities for stroke families. There are times when it is good to be able to reach out and draw on the help of others. One member explained her reason for joining a stroke club: "I've been trying to deal with this on my own for 2 years and couldn't. The hostility one time, the caring the next time—it became a battle. Therefore I'm going to counseling for myself, to learn to be me and to do interesting things in my own life and still carry on."

The long arm of stroke also affected a young man in California whose sister had moved home to North Carolina to care for their father who had a stroke: "Others don't realize the day-by-day frustrations that my sister is going through. I am out in California having a good time while my sister is caring for my father. . . . I have to live with a certain amount of guilt."

SUMMARY

It is important to be able to distinguish between the emotions and reality, and knowing that you must deal with both. By being aware of both, one can deal with the totality of the situation and keep that balance of the thinking and the emotion in one's own mind. If one tries to block out that emotion and deal simply with the reality, it is not going to work; and if one deals just with the emotions, he becomes "hung up" on that too. Tunnel vision is an ever present trap for the unwary, and the trick is to find the path in between. Stroke touches many people, and sacrifices by the family and patient are needed. Suggestions for the caregiver at home include setting goals for yourself . . . that you have a life to live as well as the patient; try to live as normal a life as possible despite demands made on your time, and do for yourself. One family member suggested that a live-in nurse was as important to her as buying food.

As one 31-year-old man, who had had a stroke when he was 25, said, "The first emotion is denial . . . this isn't really happening. Then comes anger, then frustration, then apathy. This is it. One life to live. This is my reality . . . I have no control over it. It's the way things worked out. No one I know has any control over it. No one wanted it to work out this way. . . ."

9

Motor Skills Problems

Barbara Freiberg

After a stroke, most patients need physical and/or occupational therapy to help with recovery from the effects of the stroke. Depending on the area of the brain involved, a patient may show muscle weakness, sensory loss, incoordination, decreased balance, and/or difficulty following directions and speaking. In turn, these problems interfere with one's ability to walk, communicate, and perform self-care skills such as feeding, bathing, and dressing. Often these everyday activities have to be relearned.

Therapy hastens the return of function; it helps the patient develop proper movements and habits as well as learn new ways to perform old activities. During a normal recovery most of the improvements occur within the first 3 months after a stroke, with some further improvements occurring over an additional 3-month period. A few improvements may be seen up to a year following the stroke. Usually the sooner a patient regains strength and the ability to move, the better is his prognosis for continued improvement. The extent of initial loss of muscle function is important when determining prognosis.

The purpose of this chapter is to familiarize the reader with the various aspects of the treatment program the stroke patient may encounter during physical or occupational therapy sessions. The family members or other caregivers reading it will gain an understanding of the effects therapy usually has on the recovery process of stroke patients. Appropriate exercises, walking, self-care, equipment needs, and discharge planning are addressed. The emphasis of therapy is on what the patient can do for himself and how the caregiver can help when assistance is needed.

There are some suggestions on how family members may assist patients in their care and therapy programs. Note that families should receive specific instructions from their doctors and therapists before using any of the suggestions in this section.

SENSORY CHANGES

Often the stroke patient suffers numbness or sensory changes in addition to muscle weakness. Sometimes the sensory losses are pronounced, and occasionally they are the only resulting symptom of the stroke.

With severe loss of sensation, the patient may ignore the extremities (arms and legs) on the involved side because of their profound loss of sensation. Frequently, the patient has visual problems that prevent seeing to one side, or homonymous hemianopsia. These visual problems make the sensory loss worse. With the combination of loss of sensation and visual limitations, the involved side is sometimes perceived by the patient to belong to someone else or as not existing at all. Hence such patients are taught to pay more attention to the involved side. To compensate for the decreased vision on one side, they are encouraged to turn their heads and look toward that side.

Safety is stressed to patients who have decreased sensation. Particular attention must be paid to the prevention of burns caused by hot water, space heaters, heating pads, or cigarettes. Burns may occur because of the difficulty of perceiving temperature changes. When neglect of the extremity occurs, there is an increased possibility of injury to that extremity. The extremity may be caught on or jammed by an obstacle without the patient's awareness. The patient is taught to frequently check the position of his arm or leg in order to prevent injury.

Sensory losses may affect one's coordination. Everyone has had the experience of trying to pick up an object while the hand is "asleep." Without being able to feel things normally, it becomes difficult to know where that object is in the hand or how hard it must be gripped to hold onto it.

These decreased sensations also affect the stroke patient's ability to walk. When trying to stand on a leg that feels "asleep," there is a fear that the knee will buckle. This lack of sensation also affects the ability to place the foot properly while walking. Initially, some stroke patients must watch their feet for proper placement while relearning to walk. As judgment in foot placement improves, patients are encouraged to look up while walking.

Some patients have an increased response to touch instead of a numb feeling. Such increased awareness of touch is called hypersensitivity. In such cases therapists work on reducing the sense of touch to a normal level of feeling.

Sensory disturbances can affect a patient's safety and ability to move. Such changes must be taken into consideration when working on all other aspects of the therapy program.

SKIN CARE AND BED POSITIONING

Bed sores and skin irritations can develop after a stroke if proper care is not provided. Good skin care requires frequent changes in position to prevent pressure areas or bed sores. Proper positioning of a stroke patient must be started immediately. Positioning techniques need to be followed throughout the bed-confined stage.

Generally, while bed-confined the patient's position should be changed every 2 hours. Position changes include lying on the back, the affected or involved side, and the unaffected or uninvolved side. Position changes help prevent pressure areas or bed sores by allowing the blood circulation to flow more freely as weight is shifted off a body part. Lotion can be rubbed gently on the skin if no pressure sores are present.

Pillows, towel rolls, or specially designed cushions may be used to help maintain a position or support a body part. Frequent change in limb positions also helps maintain the mobility of the joints. Proper bed positioning techniques are shown in Fig. 6.

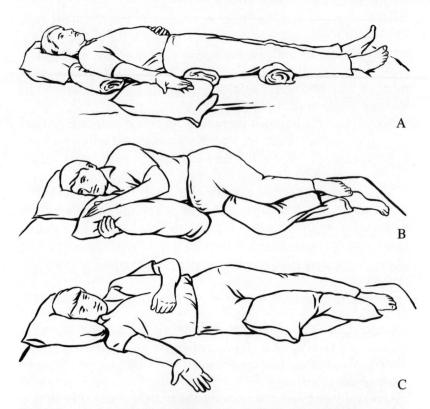

FIG. 6. A: Bed positioning. Back-lying; pillows and towel rolls are used for positioning. **B:** Side-lying on the uninvolved side. The involved shoulder and hip are forward, with the arm and leg supported on pillows. **C:** Side-lying on the involved side. The involved shoulder is forward, and the pillow is between the knees.

EATING

Before a stroke patient begins to eat or drink, a feeding tube or nasogastric tube may be needed to provide nutrients. This tube is placed through the nose and continues through the esophagus directly to the stomach. The patient is evaluated as to his ability to manage food and for safety of eating before the regular (by mouth) feeding program is initiated.

The ability to cough and clear the airway is important for determining safety during eating. The patient must be able to swallow effectively to avoid choking. Ice chips are sometimes used for testing the ability to swallow without getting the substance into the airway or the lungs.

The consistency of the food varies according to the patient's ability to chew and swallow. Difficulty in swallowing is called dysphagia. Pureed or soft foods may be easier to swallow than liquids. If that is the case, liquids may be added to the patient's diet last so as to avoid choking. Puddings, thick soups, or pureed foods may be offered first if chewing or swallowing is a problem. As soon as possible, a regular diet is recommended.

Initially, a stoke patient may need assistance while eating but should begin to feed himself as soon as possible. The patient uses his uninvolved hand to feed himself. If needed, special adaptive equipment may be provided by the occupational therapist. To allow easier eating and digesting, the patient should be in a sitting position for meals. Sitting while eating allows safer and more efficient management of the food.

When beginning to eat, the patient may need assistance guiding the spoon or fork to the dish and from the dish to the mouth. As he improves, less hands-on assistance is needed. This procedure may need to be repeated many times before the patient can initiate and complete the feeding process on his own. The food should be placed toward the uninvolved side of the mouth to allow easier swallowing. If there are sensory or motor losses in the mouth, the patient may be unaware of food on the involved side. Thus food may be lodged in the cheek and can later cause choking because the patient is unaware of its presence. Therefore it is important to check the mouth during the feeding process. Swallowing and clearing food from the involved cheek can be assisted by placing the hand on the outside of the cheek and massaging the area. Keeping the head slightly forward helps prevent food from entering the airway during swallowing.

Patients with visual involvement may have difficulty seeing the food on their involved side. They are thus encouraged to turn their heads to the involved side to compensate for their reduced field of vision.

Adaptive equipment can aid self-feeding. Plate guards or scoop dishes provide a rim around the plate to allow scooping of the food. Rocker knives can be used for cutting foods one-handedly. Also, nonskid materials used on the bottom of plates or a damp washcloth placed under the plate prevents slippage on the table.

Milk cartons can be managed by securing the container between the knees while using the uninvolved hand to open the carton. Salt, sugar, and pepper packages can be torn open using the teeth.

BATHING AND HYGIENE

The stroke patient can begin helping with his bath while still confined to the bed. Initially, he may wash his face and hands and brush his teeth or care for his dentures. It allows the patient to take part in his care and encourages him to be aware of both sides of his body. By beginning with the involved side, the patient is sure not to forget to bathe that area.

Bathing in bed or in a chair at the sink allows full concentration on the bathing activity without worrying about losing one's balance. As the patient becomes more mobile, he starts to bathe using a tub bench. The tub bench is placed within the tub or shower and allows showering while seated. Whenever possible, the patient should use a tub bench, rather than the tub itself, in order to prevent slipping or falling when getting in and out of the tub. If a patient is able to walk to the tub, he turns and sits on the tub bench before bringing his legs into the tub. To transfer from the wheelchair, the patient slides over to the tub seat and then brings his legs into the tub. A hand-held shower allows easier cleansing. Grab bars and rubber mats are placed in the shower or tub to allow safer transfers.

The occupational therapist may suggest some adaptive equipment to ease self-bathing. These devices are available commercially or can be made at home. A long-handled bath sponge can be used to bathe hard-to-reach spots. Wash mitts can be made by sewing two washcloths together. Soap on a rope eliminates reaching for a bar of soap.

Shaving is performed most easily using an electric razor but can be accomplished with a straight edge razor as well. Extra caution must be observed if using a straight edge razor. If a person is neglecting the involved side, he may need to be reminded to wash and shave that area.

Aerosol deodorant is easier to apply than the roll-on variety. The involved arm can be propped on a pillow, away from the body, for deodorant application. To apply deodorant to the involved arm, the deodorant is held in the uninvolved hand as it is sprayed.

Bedside commodes may be used if a patient is unable to get to the bathroom. Bedside commodes are available with removable armrests to ease transferring from the bed or wheelchair to the commode. If a patient can get to the bathroom, it may be helpful to use a grab bar for support and/or a raised toilet seat to extend the height of the present commode. These steps allow safer and easier toilet usage. If standing balance is decreased, men should sit to urinate.

DRESSING

Dressing activities usually are initiated after a patient can sit safely in a chair or a wheelchair. Some self-dressing can be accomplished while in bed, but the following recommendations deal with dressing in a sitting position.

Selection of clothing is important. Sleeping attire may be used during early recovery, but the wearing of street clothes should be encouraged as soon as possible. Comfortable, loose-fitting clothes are recommended. Front-opening tops or dresses and T-shirts are most convenient. For women half-slips and brassieres that fasten in the front are easier to manage. If buttons and zippers are difficult to fasten, Velcro closures can be substituted. Velcro is available at most fabric shops, and some clothes and shoes are made with Velcro fasteners. These items may be ordered through some specialty catalogs that carry assistive devices and clothing for the physically impaired.

When dressing, the patient is seated in an armchair or a locked wheelchair. Following are directions and diagrams for self-dressing.

Putting on a Front-Opening Shirt: Method I

1. The shirt is positioned on the patient's lap (Fig. 7). The label is facing up with the collar toward his knees. The armhole for the involved arm is spread open. The patient uses his uninvolved arm to pick up the involved arm. He reaches across the shirt and places the involved arm into the appropriate sleeve.
2. The sleeve is pulled up over the elbow and up to the armpit (Fig. 8).
3. The shirt is pulled over the involved shoulder and around the back. The uninvolved arm is slipped into the correct armhole (Fig. 9).
4. The patient leans slightly forward and pulls the shirt down in the back. The shirt is properly adjusted and the buttons fastened (Fig. 10).

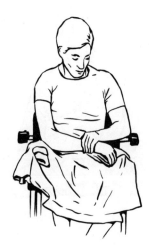

FIG. 7. The shirt is on the patient's lap, with the label facing up and the collar toward the knees. The uninvolved hand reaches across to place the involved arm in the appropriate sleeve.

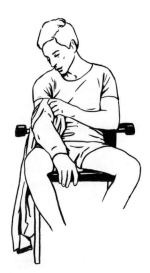

FIG. 8. The sleeve is pulled up to the armpit on the involved arm.

FIG. 9. The shirt is pulled up over the involved shoulder and around the back. The uninvolved arm is slipped into the correct armhole.

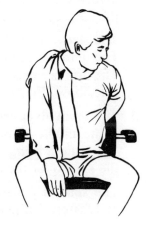

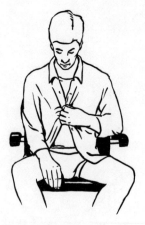

FIG. 10. The shirt is pulled down in the back and properly adjusted.

Putting on a Front-Opening Shirt or T-shirt: Method II

1. The shirt is positioned on the patient's lap. The label is facing up with the collar toward his chest. The sleeve for the involved arm is spread open. The patient uses his uninvolved arm to pick up the involved arm and place it in the sleeve opening (Fig. 11).

2. The sleeve is pulled up over the elbow and to the armpit. The uninvolved arm is slipped into the appropriate sleeve. The arm is raised and the sleeve slipped into position past the elbow (Fig. 12).

3. The uninvolved hand gathers the shirt from hem to collar in the middle of the back. The shirt is raised over the head. The patient brings his head down and leans forward to slip the shirt over the head (Fig. 13).

4. The shirt is pulled down in the back, properly adjusted, and fastened if needed (Fig. 14).

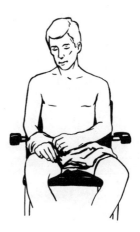

FIG. 11. The shirt is on the patient's lap with the label facing up and the collar toward the chest. The uninvolved hand helps place the involved arm into the sleeve opening.

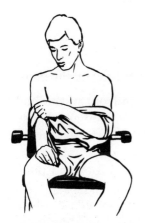

FIG. 12. The sleeves are pulled up past the elbows—involved arm first.

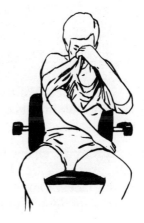

FIG. 13. The uninvolved hand gathers the shirt from hem to collar in the back, and the patient slips it over his head.

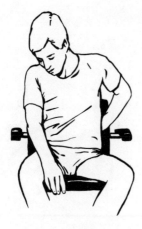

FIG. 14. The shirt is pulled down in the back and properly adjusted.

Putting on Pants

The belt is put through the loops before putting on the pants.

1. The uninvolved leg is placed directly in front of the body with the foot flat on the floor. The uninvolved arm is used to pick up the involved leg and place it over the uninvolved leg in a crossed-leg position (Fig. 15).
2. The pant leg is slipped over the involved foot and pulled up to the knee (Fig. 16).
3. The involved leg is uncrossed and the foot gently placed on the floor. The uninvolved leg is placed into the pants. The pants are pulled up as far as possible (Fig. 17).
4. The patient now stands and completes pulling the pants up to the waist (Fig. 18). Be sure the pants are not caught under either heel before standing.
5. The patient sits down. The pants and belt are fastened (Fig. 19).

It may be easier to wear shoes that slip on or have Velcro closures. Elastic laces are available to eliminate the need for tying laces. One-handed tying of laces can be learned by the stroke patient who prefers to continue using standard laces.

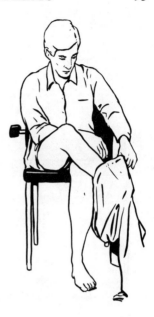

FIG. 15. The involved leg is crossed over the uninvolved leg.

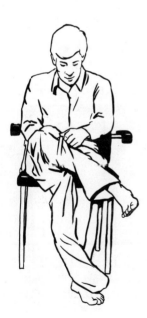

FIG. 16. The pant leg is slipped over the involved foot and pulled up to the knee.

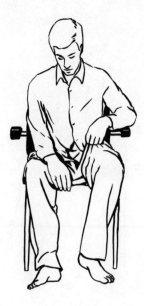

FIG. 17. The uninvolved leg is placed into the pants, and the pants are pulled up as far as possible.

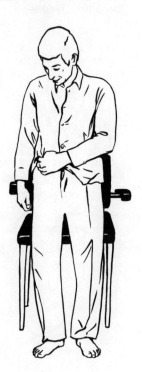

FIG. 18. While standing, the pants are pulled up to the waist.

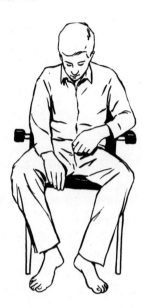

FIG. 19. While sitting, the pants are fastened.

Assistive devices such as reachers and dressing sticks are used when patients have limitations in their reach capability. These devices help pick up objects of clothing and pull clothes up into place. Button hooks may be used to ease fastening buttons.

There are many more devices available commercially or easily constructed at home. The therapist working with the patient can offer suggestions concerning assistive devices. Whenever possible the patient is taught how to dress without the use of such devices, but occasionally these aids are needed to provide independence in self-care.

GETTING OUT OF BED

After the stroke patient is medically stable, the physician recommends that the patient begin to engage in activities out of bed. The nurses or therapists assist the patient to a sitting position. The amount of time spent sitting depends on the patient's condition and his ability to tolerate this new position. Generally, the first session lasts about one-half hour. Blood pressure monitoring may be used to determine one's tolerance to sitting.

Initially, patients may need to be lifted into and out of the bed or chair. Moving from one area to another, as from bed to chair, is called transferring. As early as possible, the patient is instructed to assist in the transfer. The chair is placed so that the front corner touches the bed and is positioned at a slight angle with the bed instead of being directly side by side. Figures 20 to 23 demonstrate transferring from a bed to a wheelchair.

If possible, the armrest of the wheelchair closest to the bed is removed. Many therapists teach transferring toward the patient's uninvolved or strongest side, although there are some advocates of transferring toward the involved or weaker side. In most cases patients need to be able to transfer toward either side prior to being discharged. The proper transfer method is recommended based on the therapist's evaluation of the patient's needs and abilities.

If equipment with wheels is being used, be sure to lock all brakes. Properly place the equipment and instruct the patient as to what he needs to do during the transfer. Always use safe and proper body mechanics. The person helping in the transfer should lift by bending at the knees instead of the back. The patient is taught to pivot on his feet as he moves toward the new position.

The same principles are to be used for transfers between any two surfaces, such as from wheelchairs to tub seats, commodes, or cars. Always be sure to explain to the patient how you will be performing the transfer and what you expect him to do to help. Be consistent with your directions and transfer technique. Have the patient wear shoes with nonskid bottoms to avoid slipping during the transfer.

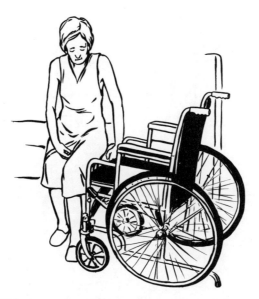

FIG. 20. The patient pushes up from the bed.

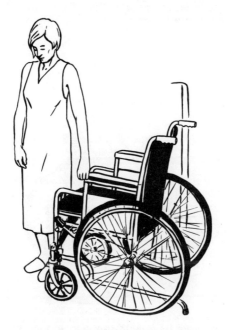

FIG. 21. After standing, the patient turns and reaches for the further-most armrest.

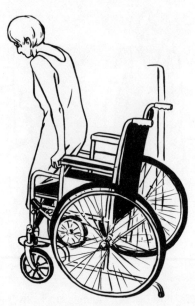

FIG. 22. With the back of the legs close to or touching the chair, the patient holds onto the armrest.

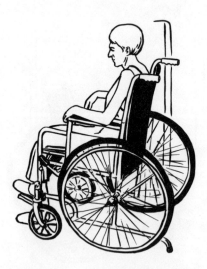

FIG. 23. The patient sits with the involved leg on the footrest.

EXERCISE

After a stroke a patient must begin an exercise program as soon as possible. Exercises are important for preventing complications caused by immobility and for strengthening weak muscles. Range of motion exercises help prevent the formation of blood clots (which may form because of slowed circulation associated with a decrease in muscle movements). Exercises are also important for maintaining mobility in the joints and preventing muscle tightening. If exercises are not performed, joint contractures can develop. Contractures are stiff joints caused by shortening of muscles and ligaments after prolonged immobility. Once a contracture develops, intensive exercising or surgery is required to improve the motion in the joint.

An exercise program may be started before the patient begins getting out of bed and continues even after discharge from the hospital. The therapists and nurses assist the patient with the exercises and may teach the family how to do them. If the patient is unable to assist in performing the exercises, the program is called passive range of motion. Attempts to encourage muscle functioning are initiated by the therapy team and adjusted as the patient improves. As the patient participates more in his rehabilitation, he may be taught to exercise on his own. As strength returns, resistance may be applied manually or mechanically to further increase muscle strength.

Usually weakness is limited to one side and is called hemiparesis or hemiplegia. Improvement in the use of the involved leg usually precedes improvement in the use of the involved arm. Often return of movement is seen last in the hand and ankle muscles. The amount of improvement possible varies, but few patients recover completely from a stroke.

Patients who are beginning to get some return of movement in their arm often maintain a position of flexion involuntarily.

It is seen as a balling up of fingers into a fist and bending of the elbow. Because this position is maintained for long periods of time, it is important to exercise the joints to the opposite position with the fingers and elbow straight. Squeezing a ball is not recommended because it encourages too much flexion.

Another area of the arm that needs particular attention is the shoulder joint. If exercises are not performed often enough or incorrectly, the shoulder can become painful during any motion. Proper exercise early and throughout the rehabilitation program can help prevent this problem. If the shoulder does become painful, exercises must be gentle and limited to avoid increasing pain.

The leg is less likely to develop areas of pain, but joint stiffness can develop if the exercises are not performed regularly and properly. The ankle joint needs frequent stretching to prevent tightening of the calf muscle.

An exercise program for stroke patients is shown in Figs. 24 through 49. Generally, each exercise is repeated 5 to 10 times once or twice a day. The therapist treating the stroke patient discusses any special considerations or precautions to be observed with the caregiver.

Some electrical devices are used to help encourage muscle functioning. The most frequently used devices are vibrators, biofeedback machines, and muscle stimulators. Vibrators rubbed over muscles cause involuntary movements. Some therapists think that return of voluntary movement is hastened by using the vibrator. Biofeedback machines use a blinking light or a buzzing sound to indicate the functioning of a muscle. This method provides the patient with a mechanism for knowing if the muscle is working, and it encourages stronger muscle responses. Electrical stimulators use electrical current to make muscles function involuntarily in hopes of encouraging voluntary function.

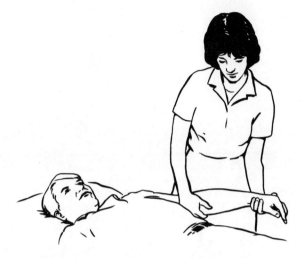

FIG. 24. Supporting the wrist and elbow.

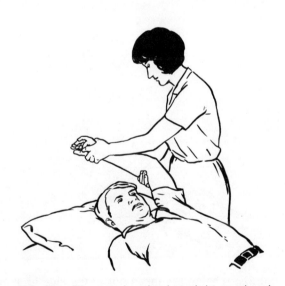

FIG. 25. The arm is raised straight overhead.

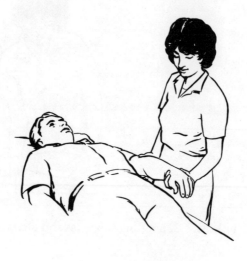

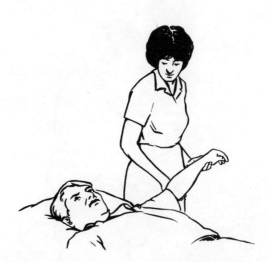

FIGS. 26 and **27.** The arm is taken out to the side to shoulder level while being supported at the wrist and elbow.

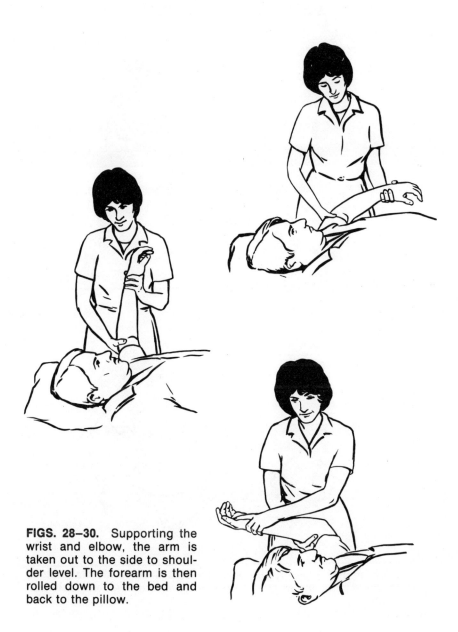

FIGS. 28–30. Supporting the wrist and elbow, the arm is taken out to the side to shoulder level. The forearm is then rolled down to the bed and back to the pillow.

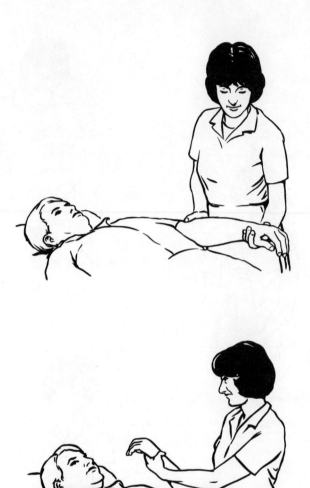

FIGS. 31 and **32.**   Giving support to the wrist, the elbow is straightened, with the palm facing the bed, and then bent, with the palm facing the shoulder.

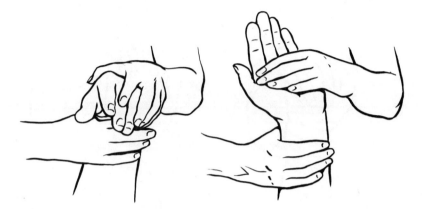

FIGS. 33 and **34.** Holding the hand and supporting it below the wrist, bend the wrist down and up.

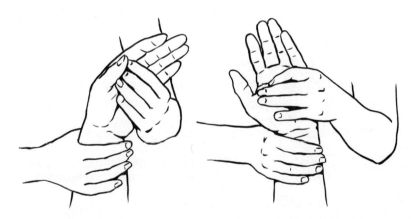

FIGS. 35 and **36.** Bend the wrist from side to side.

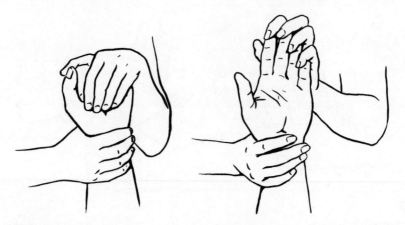

FIGS. 37 and **38.** Giving support to the wrist, bend and straighten each finger.

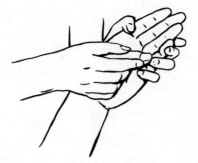

FIG. 39. Bend the thumb toward the little finger and then stretch it away from the hand.

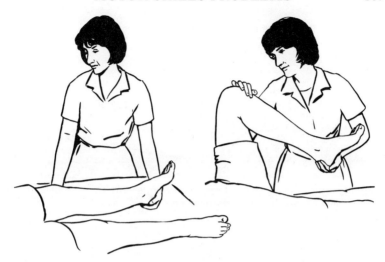

FIGS. 40 and **41.** Giving support at the heel and knee, bend the knee toward the chest and then straighten the leg back out.

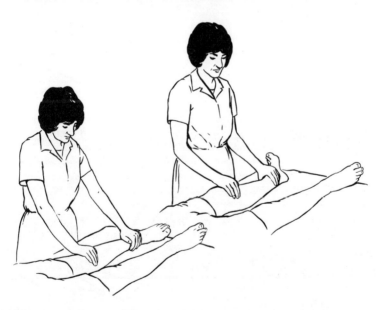

FIGS. 42 and **43.** Holding the patient at the knee and ankle, roll the leg in and out.

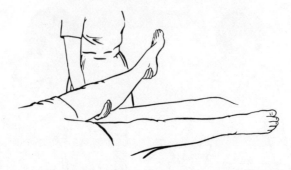

FIG. 44. Supporting the patient at the knee and ankle, move the leg out to the side and back to the middle.

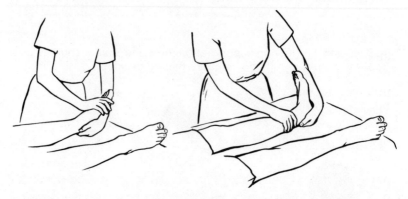

FIGS. 45 and **46.** Holding the heel with your hand and resting the foot on your forearm, bend the foot up and down at the ankle.

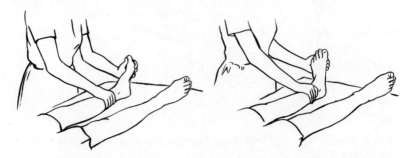

FIGS. 47 and **48.** Turn the forefoot from side to side.

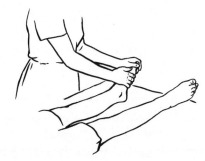

FIG. 49. Bend and straighten the toes.

BALANCE ACTIVITIES

Before beginning to walk, the stroke patient must develop good sitting and standing balance. Often the patient loses his balance while sitting because the weak trunk muscles on the involved side are unable to prevent the trunk from leaning. Patients may fall sideward, forward, or backward because of the trunk weakness. Close supervision may be needed to prevent falling and to help overcome the fear of falling.

The therapist works with the stroke patient to strengthen both abdominal and back muscles in order to increase the patient's ability to sit upright. Often it is helpful to use a mirror in front of the patient to allow visual cueing. The visual cues help the stroke patient realize what the upright posture feels like. Because of numbness or sensory losses on the involved side, the stroke patient may have difficulty knowing if he is sitting straight.

Strengthening exercises may involve having the patient push against the therapist toward different directions. Another method to strengthen the trunk muscles is to have the patient hold an upright position while the therapist gently pushes against the patient. These same activities can be applied in the standing position. The therapist gently pushes against the patient to strengthen trunk muscles and to assist the patient in regaining his ability to balance in the standing position.

Weight-shifting activities are often emphasized while standing, and sometimes while sitting, to encourage the patient to
bear weight over his involved or weakened leg. Because of
weakness, sensory losses, and fear the patient often avoids
using the weak leg when standing. Such avoidance causes all
of the patient's weight to be distributed over the stronger or
uninvolved leg. If this habit is not corrected before walking
begins, the patient continues to have difficulty standing on the
weak leg and favors the stronger leg. Once balance is achieved
in a stationary position, the patient needs to work on maintaining his balance while walking.

WALKING

The total process for safe walking or ambulation involves
coming to the standing position, balancing while standing,
walking a distance, and returning to the sitting position. To
assume the standing position, the patient is taught to move to
the front edge of the chair. The feet are placed so that as the
person leans forward to rise out of the chair his weight is
directly over his feet. Often patients need to be reminded to
bring the involved leg back to help support the body weight.
The uninvolved hand pushes on the armrest of the chair to
help the patient stand up from the chair.

Walking usually begins by standing in the parallel bars. Parallel bars are a set of secure horizontal bars the patient can
grasp for support. Good standing balance and the ability to
shift the body weight from one leg to the other are essential
before a patient can safely walk. Initially, the therapist may
assist the patient in bringing the weak leg forward. It may be
necessary for the therapist to manually support the knee to
prevent it from buckling as the patient bears weight on the
weak leg. With practice and with return of function, the patient
improves his ability to advance and control the involved leg.
The therapist or helper gives help only as needed. It is important not to let the patient lean on the helper or become too
dependent on his assistance.

As ambulation improves, the therapist encourages the patient to walk outside the parallel bars. At this point the patient should be able to advance his weak leg, support his body weight, and shift his weight onto the weak leg as he advances his stronger leg.

Some patients require the use of a foot brace or an assistive device such as a cane. There are several types of canes available. Braces and assistive devices, along with other equipment needs, are discussed later in this chapter.

To return to the sitting position, the patient backs up to the chair until his legs are touching or are close to the front of the seat. Before sitting, the patient reaches for the armrest of his chair with the uninvolved hand. This move ensures that he is in the correct position, helps prevent the chair from moving, and allows him to gently lower himself into the chair.

Usually, stair climbing instructions encourage leading with the uninvolved leg as the patient goes up the stairs. To go down the stairs, the involved leg leads. Stairs are handled one at a time. As a patient improves his ability to go up and down stairs, he returns to the normal pattern of taking each stair with an alternating leg. Using handrails provides safety and stability. If a cane is used, the cane remains on the same step as the involved leg.

Walking on carpets can be more difficult than walking on linoleum or tile floors. The involved leg must be lifted higher to prevent tripping while walking on carpets. Throw rugs should be removed from the home environment to prevent slipping or tripping on them.

It is advisable to always wear regular shoes and not house slippers when walking. The therapist can give advice about the selection of safe footwear.

A belt around the patient's waist may be used by the therapist or helper to ensure safety while walking. The belt allows assistance to be provided in case of balance difficulties without grabbing the patient's arm. It is important not to provide more support than the patient needs.

EQUIPMENT NEEDS

Some patients need special equipment after suffering a stroke. Following are several commonly used devices.

Splints

Hand splints may be fitted to the stroke patient to maintain proper hand positioning. These splints are usually made of plastic. The hand is functionally positioned so the wrist is slightly extended; the fingers are bent at the knuckles and straight in the digits. The thumb is positioned comfortably away from the fingers. Wearing time and proper care of the splints are discussed by the therapy staff working with the stroke patient. Some therapists prefer using a cone or cylinder placed in the patient's palm to position the hand.

Arm Slings or Arm Trays

Support in the form of a sling or tray may be provided for the involved arm. This device protects the hemiplegic arm and provides support at the shoulder, helping to prevent subluxation of the shoulder joint. Without support, the weight of the arm can cause stretching of the structures in the shoulder joint or subluxation. Subluxation is defined as separation of the bone of the upper arm from the shoulder. It results in a painful shoulder. Once subluxation occurs, it cannot be corrected. Generally, slings are used while the arm is paralyzed, but they may be discarded if function returns. There are many types of slings available, and the therapist working with the stroke patient can recommend the appropriate one. Instead of slings, arm trays or lap boards may be attached to the wheelchair for support of the involved arm. Such a support allows the arm to be elevated for management of swelling and places the hand in a visible position. With the arm supported and visible, the patient is encouraged to touch and exercise it.

Leg Braces

Weakness of the ankle muscles can cause dragging of the toes or foot while walking. Foot splints or braces substitute for the weakened ankle muscles. These devices provide proper ankle positioning and support, and allow safer walking. Splints are made of plastic and fit inside the shoe. Braces are made of metal uprights that clamp into a channel fitted into the heel of the shoe. The braces have an ankle joint, which allows some ankle motion and ensures correct positioning of the ankle while walking. Splints and braces reduce the chance of tripping caused by toe dragging.

Walkers and Canes

Walkers are used if the main problem of walking is poor balance or ataxia. The walker provides more support when lack of balance interferes with safe walking. Both arms are needed for handling a walker.

For patients whose stroke has caused one-sided weakness or hemiparesis, a cane may be used while walking. It is held in the uninvolved hand. The therapist working with the stroke patient can help select the appropriate cane.

There are canes that have three or four legs for a base of support. These devices are called hemicanes, pyramid canes, quad canes, or tripod canes, depending on the design. Standard canes may be used if a patient has better balance and improved function of the involved leg.

Wheelchairs

Wheelchairs may be needed if a patient is not capable of walking safely on his own. Using a wheelchair can help gain some independence. The physical therapist can give advice when selecting a wheelchair. Options include removable armrests, removable footrests, elevating legrests, and one-arm drive. Chairs are available in different sizes and need to be selected to properly accommodate each person.

Wheelchairs can be rented or purchased, depending on one's needs. In some communities, organizations loan equipment.

DISCHARGE FROM THE HOSPITAL

Prior to the patient's discharge from the hospital, family members or primary caregivers are encouraged to come to the hospital for home instructions. The nurses and therapists outline a program to meet the individual patient's needs. Emphasis is placed on what the patient can do for himself and on how the caregiver can help when assistance is needed.

The home program may include bed positioning, exercising, walking, and performing self-care skills. An opportunity is provided for demonstrating and practicing these activities. If special equipment or home modifications are needed, recommendations are made by the staff.

If further therapy is needed after being discharged from the hospital, arrangements can be made for a therapist to come to the home or the patient can return to a hospital or an outpatient clinic for follow-up care. The frequency of therapy depends on the individual's needs and on what services are available in the community. It is helpful to keep on record the phone number of the therapist who reviewed the home instructions in case questions or problems arise at a later date.

MODIFICATIONS IN THE HOME ENVIRONMENT

Modifications to the entrance of the house and within the interior of the house may be necessary for safety and optimal independence for a stroke patient. Stairs, doorways, furniture, and cabinets may require alterations to accommodate a wheelchair or an ambulatory stroke patient. There are many assistive devices and pieces of adaptive equipment available to simplify homemaking skills and bathroom needs. Suggestions concerning home modifications are discussed in Chapter 10.

DRIVING

Returning to driving a car requires good strength, perceptual skills, vision, coordination, and reflexes. The physician and therapist can advise the patient when he is ready to drive a vehicle. Anyone who has had a stroke and is considering driving again needs to be retested at the state's Department of Motor Vehicles. Driver's licenses must be reissued after any major illness or accident that has resulted in physical or psychological impairment.

RETURNING TO WORK AND LEISURE ACTIVITIES

Many patients and family members ask when the stroke patient will be able to return to work. Generally, the patient's doctor can give advice as to if or when it will be possible to resume working.

Factors to be considered are the amount of physical and psychological impairment caused by the stroke and the type of work required by the job. The decision regarding the return to work must be made on an individual basis.

The employer's cooperation in modifying schedules or job descriptions is helpful. Sometimes a person initially returns on a part-time basis. It might also be necessary to change the job requirements so as to avoid tasks that are too difficult but to emphasize other skills and abilities of the employee. Sometimes changes in the work environment are needed for safety reasons.

If it is not possible to return to one's old job, it may be possible to look into other jobs or alternatives. Vocational counselors can evaluate the stroke person's abilities for employment. Vocational rehabilitation departments are available in many communities to provide such assistance. Such offices are federally and state funded. People are evaluated by counselors to determine eligibility for vocational rehabilitation services.

For people who cannot return to a paying job, volunteer jobs or hobbies may be rewarding. People who were employed outside the home may assume new responsibilities in the home as an alternative. This switching of responsibilities may allow another family member to work outside the home.

Recreational therapists help stroke patients adapt old hobbies to their current capabilities or learn new leisure activities. The recreational therapist can also help in the transition of returning to the community after hospitalization.

SUMMARY

The physical and occupational therapy information presented covers some of the basic concerns and considerations of the rehabilitation of the stroke patient. Patients and family members should use these suggestions as a guide. It is important to remember that each patient is different and so has different needs. A therapist can evaluate a stroke patient and then provide a thorough treatment program. The information provided here covers only some treatment procedures and a sampling of equipment and assistive devices available.

Increasing one's understanding of the stroke process and the rationale and goals of treatment makes it easier to cope with this significant change in life style. Further information dealing with physical and occupational therapy concerns may be found by referring to one of the following resource books or pamphlets.

Therapy

Home Care for the Stroke Patient, by M. Johnstone, 1978. Available from Churchill Livingstone, 1560 Broadway, New York, NY 10036.

Accessibility Design

The System. Available from Information Development Corporation, 360 St. Alban Court, Winston-Salem, NC 27103.

An Illustrated Handbook of the Handicapped Section of the North Carolina State Building Code, Special Office for the Handicapped. Available from the North Carolina Department of Insurance, P.O. Box 26387, Raleigh, NC 27611.

Accessibility Modifications: Guidelines for Modifications to Existing Buildings for Accessibility. Available from the North Carolina Department of Insurance, P.O. Box 26387, Raleigh, NC 27611.

Accessible Housing. Available from the North Carolina Department of Insurance, P.O. Box 26387, Raleigh, NC 27611.

Adaptive Equipment

The Capability Collection. Available from Ways & Means, 28001 Citrin Drive, Romulus, MI 48174.

Common Problems, Useful Solutions after a Stroke. Available from AliMedina, 297 High Street, Dedham, MA 02026.

Enrichments—Catalog for Better Living. Available from Bissell Healthcare Companies, P.O. Box 579, Hinsdale, IL 60521.

Sears Home Health Care Catalog. Available from Sears, Roebuck and Co., Sears Tower, Chicago, IL 60684.

Professional Health Care Catalog. Available from Fred Sammons, Inc., P.O. 32, Brookfield, IL 60513.

Comfortably Yours—Aids for Easier Living. Available from Comfortably Yours, 52 West Hunter Avenue, Maywood, NJ 07607.

10

Home Modifications

Ronald L. Mace

Many changes in the home can be made and may be necessary to allow the individual who has had a stroke to be independent, safe, and comfortable at home. The changes range from the simple addition of a piece of hardware to extensive renovations or a unique, innovative adaptation of a piece of equipment. An abundance of special products and equipment are available through special sources, such as durable medical equipment dealers and mail order catalogs. However, most home modifications can be accomplished with standard hardware and building materials available from local supply companies.

It is usually best to make permanent modifications that work well for the entire family, look ordinary, and do not damage the resale value of the home. With good information and careful planning, such changes can often be made inexpensively and need not make the house look "clinical."

ENTRANCES

Getting in and out of most homes can be difficult and dangerous for anyone with a mobility impairment. Steps and stairs at entrances probably need some modification. Adding handrails may be all that is required for the post-stroke person who can go up and down stairs. For those who cannot, a ramp may be best. Ramps must not be steeper than a 1 inch vertical rise

118

in 12 inches of length and, in fact, should be flatter if possible. Wood ramps are least expensive, but they do have to be replaced periodically. Masonry and concrete ramps are more expensive but permanent. Handrails, snow removal, and waterproofing are safety and maintenance issues that must be considered. If the family does not own the home, it may be best to consider one of several prefabricated metal or fiberglass ramp systems that can be assembled or disassembled and therefore taken if the family moves. Another attractive solution, where space permits, is to terrace up the entrance with earth, creating a sloping sidewalk and a short bridge over to the house. With proper planting this earth berm becomes a garden that enhances the appearance of any home.

DOORS

Door widths may be too narrow for a person using a wheelchair or a walker. Doors can be widened but require major structural renovation of the walls. Before going to that expense, it may be best to try installing special swing-free hinges that move the door out of the opening as they swing. These hinges give up to 2 inches more clear width. If that is not enough, renovation may be the only answer.

A small loop handle installed on the pull side of a door near the hinge edge can make it easy for a mobility-impaired person to pull a door closed.

High thresholds may have to be removed or have small ramps installed on each side so wheels can easily roll over them.

For people who have extreme difficulty with doors, motorized door operators are available for both swinging and sliding residential doors. They can be installed without structural renovation.

Some people are unable to grasp and hold smooth doorknobs. Add-on lever handles in plastic and metal are available in materials and colors to match existing hardware. These handles clamp onto existing knobs and allow one to open the door without gripping.

KITCHENS

Kitchens present numerous problems, but most can be eliminated or alternatives found. Wheelchair users and people who cannot stand for long periods find the standard 36-inch kitchen counters too high. A lowered portion of the counter, a separate low table, or a rolling cart can be installed to provide a comfortable food preparation surface. This surface must have knee space underneath to allow a seated person to pull up to it.

Sinks and stoves are often too high, and the controls are frequently out of reach or difficult to operate. Special kitchen units that can be easily adjusted to any height are available, but they are quite specialized and can be expensive. Cook tops, sinks, and drop-in ranges can be installed in low cabinets or in counters with knee spaces.

When choosing appliances, try to find those with up-front controls that are easy to reach and manipulate. Devices are available that help someone with weak hands to operate stove controls. At sinks, placing or moving the faucets to the side of the sink instead of behind it may be considered. Also, faucets with lever handles are easier for everyone to use.

Overhead freezers on some refrigerators may be too high for some people who use wheelchairs or who cannot reach. Side-by-side refrigerator/freezers provide freezer and refrigerator space at all heights. Through-the-door ice and water dispensers can also help people with limited use of their hands.

Drawer pulls in the kitchen are often hidden or small and difficult to grasp. Readily available, attractive loop handles can render them usable by a person who has limited hand function.

Myriad adaptive devices are available to help someone with a mobility impairment to be independent in the kitchen. These devices are found in special mail order catalogs, and some are available through medical equipment dealers. Others, however, such as bread slicers and one-handed jar openers, are helpful for everyone and are sold widely in kitchen equipment and department stores.

COMBINING MODIFICATIONS AND ADAPTED EQUIPMENT

A combination of modifications and adapted equipment may be needed to create a kitchen that meets a disabled person's needs and is also attractive and comfortable for others to use. In any new or renovated kitchen convenience appliances such as dishwashers, disposals, and trash compactors should be considered necessities for some mobility-impaired people. When renovating a kitchen is too expensive, alternative appliances such as toaster ovens, hot plates, or microwave ovens placed in convenient locations can provide some independence.

BATHROOMS

The bathroom is another essential space in the home where some changes may be needed. Most typical residential bathrooms are too crowded to accommodate a person in a wheelchair or one who uses a walker, and the fixtures, floor covering, and controls can be hazardous.

Grab Bars

For safety and balance, grab bars may be needed at the toilet and the tub. Grab bars are now available in a range of colors and materials so they can be coordinated with other colors and avoid the institutional appearance of chrome or stainless steel. It is essential that grab bars be screwed securely to the wood studs in the wall or anchor-bolted to the structural part of the wall.

Maneuvering Space

Providing adequate maneuvering space for wheelchairs or walkers in existing bathrooms is often difficult and sometimes requires remodeling the room or relocating plumbing fixtures. At times, however, enough space can be found without major remodeling. For example, if a bathroom has a vanity lavatory cabinet, it can sometimes be replaced with a wall-hung counter and lavatory so the knee space below provides additional turning space for a person in a wheelchair.

Installing a roll-in shower sometimes solves the maneuvering space problem. For example, the tub can be removed, the bathroom floor can be waterproofed and tiled to form a roll-in shower, and the increased floor space can be used for maneuvering a wheelchair when the shower is not in use.

Toilets

Toilet seats may be too low for some post-stroke people who have difficulty rising to their feet from a low seat. Thick seats can be added to the toilet, or a spacer ring can be installed under the existing seat to raise it an inch or more. Some people benefit from toilet seats having support bars mounted on each side like arm rests. These bars are a help to many older and walking disabled people who have difficulty sitting down and getting back up again. These seats with integral bars are generally not good for wheelchair users because the enclosing bars interfere with transfers from wheelchair to toilet seat.

Bathing

Bathing is often difficult for people with mobility impairments or other physical limitations. The standard bathtub, recognized as relatively unsafe for everyone, may be unusable and hazardous for a disabled person. Products that make tubs safer and more usable include tub seats, grab bars, and non-skid materials.

Seats that fit in tubs, span the rim, or clamp to the rim allow a person to sit down outside the tub, transfer their legs over the rim, and slide into the tub area where they can remain seated at chair height while bathing. Tub seats do not work on tubs with sliding glass doors, and most require that shower curtains be cut to fit over the seat.

Typical residential stall showers do not work well for people who cannot step over their curbs and stand up while showering. The transfer shower is a bathing option for such people. These 3 × 3 foot showers are available with seats in them and are useful for many people who cannot get in tubs or stand to shower but who can transfer onto the seat. They can be conventionally built and equipped with folding seats so they can be used by a person who is either seated or standing. Plastic versions can be purchased with molded, fixed seats.

Roll-in showers are another option for bathing. They are large, open, waterproof areas where one can bathe while sitting in a special corrosion-resistant wheelchair. They have no curbs, and they can be built with tile or purchased ready-made in fiberglass and acrylic materials from several manufacturers. *Caution*: Manufactured shower stalls are large, and one-piece models do not go through doorways; therefore when remodeling, an outside wall may have to be opened in order to install them.

Grab bars are essential at tubs and showers to help people transfer and maintain balance. Single lever controls for water are easy to operate, and hand-held shower heads are useful for those who bathe while seated.

SAFETY, CONVENIENCE, AND COMFORT

Fire safety should not be overlooked when adapting a home. More than one entrance should be made accessible and usable so there is more than one way out in case of fire. Equipment and furniture must not be allowed to block exits or windows.

Electronics are now making home adaptations easy and

more effective. For example, inexpensive, battery-operated smoke detectors give early warning of fire and so provide more time for a person to react. Environmental control systems sold as security equipment now allow the control of lights, appliances, and other equipment throughout the house, or of items that are out of reach, using small key pads at one location or a remote hand-held control. These systems can be used from a bed or wheelchair. Portable telephones can be moved to any place in the house and allow the individual to receive calls or call for assistance at any time. These relatively inexpensive devices can greatly increase independence and convenience. They simply plug in and require no other installation. Note, however, that the equipment mentioned here is for the general consumer and may not be reliable enough to control critical life support systems. Fail-safe environmental control systems are available for such critical use but at much higher cost.

FURNISHINGS

Furniture can also be a benefit or a hazard to one with a disability and may need some alteration or replacement. Beds are often too high or too low to be used easily. Low beds can be raised by placing them on a wood platform. Legs can be cut off to lower those that are too high.

Carpets, if used, must have their edges secured to the floor. Throw rugs are dangerous tripping or slipping hazards and should be removed.

Chairs may also be too low and therefore make it difficult for some people to return to a standing position. Chairs with high average seat heights of 18 to 19 inches and firm cushions are best. Several manufacturers produce elevating upholstered chairs which have seats that rise electrically to help a person sit down and get back up. Available in different styles and upholstered in various fabrics, the chairs look like other, regular furniture.

Home modifications and selection of adaptive equipment

can enhance rather than detract from the appearance and value of the home. Research into options available and careful selection result in an optimum design at low cost usable by everyone and attractive to look at. Just because there is a disability, one need not build a clinic to live in.

EDITOR'S NOTE

The information in this chapter was provided by nationally known architect Ronald L. Mace, AIA, president of Barrier Free Environments, Inc. (BFE). BFE is an architectural and product design firm that specializes in designing buildings and products that are usable by everyone, including disabled and nondisabled people. The firm's architectural work includes planning both renovations and new construction for residential and commercial buildings. Its services include, but are not limited to, developing the original design and preparing complete construction drawings. If the client desires, the firm also advises on appropriate equipment and furnishings and oversees construction of the project. The firm conducts market and design research on the fit between people and the products and buildings they use.

BFE has been at the forefront of accessible design for the past 14 years. For answers to specific access problems with home design or modifications, Mr. Mace may be contacted at:

Barrier Free Environments, Inc.
P.O. Box 30634
Water Garden, Highway 70 West
Raleigh, NC 27622
(919) 782-7823

11

Language and Speech Problems

Claire Matthews

Speech and other communication problems may seem of secondary importance during the first days or weeks following the stroke, but once the initial shock and anxiety have subsided patient, family, and friends begin to recognize that one of their strongest links has weakened—their ability to communicate effectively with one another. The range of possible communication disorders is broad and includes mild slurring of speech, irrelevance, repeated utterances of one or two words, and an inability to speak at all. Nearly all stroke patients have some difficulty recalling words and some difficulty understanding what is said to them, even though this may be minimal. Whatever problems they may have understanding and producing speech are usually duplicated in their reading and writing abilities. Some patients, however, may have a reading disorder that is disproportionately severe relative to the oral language disorder.

The nature of the communication disorder influences the type of therapy selected by the speech/language pathologist. Before discussing the roles of the therapist, the family, and the patient in the rehabilitation of speech and language disorders, then, it may be helpful to review some of the disorders that may occur following stroke.

IMPAIRED COMPREHENSION

Some patients do not seem to understand all of what is said. When a stroke patient answers questions inappropriately or does not follow commands well, if at all, the assumption is that he did not understand the question or the command. These "auditory comprehension" problems may have a number of causes.

Rarely, a stroke patient is able to hear "something" but he cannot recognize what he hears. For example, doorbells, barking dogs, car horns, bird songs, and human speech all sound alike to him. He behaves as if he were deaf. The technical name for this condition is auditory agnosia. Obviously, if a person does not even recognize that the noise he is hearing is speech, he cannot be expected to understand what is being said. The language system in these rare cases is usually relatively intact. These patients can usually read well. They frequently learn to lip-read, and their speech is understandable, so communication is not terribly difficult so long as eye contact is maintained. Telephone communication, of course, is impossible.

Another source of "comprehension" problems is the inability to focus and maintain attention, to concentrate. Patients with attentional problems are easily distracted and may even seem not to remember what is expected of them from one moment to the next. Nearly everyone with brain damage has trouble attending or concentrating to some degree, particularly in noisy environments, but there are some patients whose primary problem seems to be one of attention. Patients who cannot pay attention truly *cannot*: The problem is caused by the nature of the brain damage and not by stubbornness or laziness, no matter how it may appear. Naturally, if a patient's brain forces him to pay as much attention to inconsequential noises around him as to the person who is talking to him, he cannot be expected to hear all of the message. When they are able to attend, these patients often show that they understand speech quite well, and their language may be remarkably well retained.

Another source of "comprehension" difficulties is a reduction in short-term or working memory. Again, this happens to nearly all brain-damaged patients to some degree, but there are some who are particularly afflicted. Such a patient seems to forget everything but the first (or the last) thing that was said to him, for example, in a list of instructions. Again, this problem is a function of the brain damage and not of the patient's will. Family and friends must learn ways to get around the problem. In many cases the patient understands what is said to him as it is being said but cannot retain more than one or two elements of the message for more than a second or two.

Problems in decoding the message—in actually understanding the form of the language as it is being spoken to the patient—are limited to patients whose strokes were in the left side of the brain, or occasionally in left-handed patients whose strokes were in the right side of the brain. Such patients become "aphasic": Their ability to process and produce language is impaired. Language is multifaceted, however, and more than one thing can go wrong in an aphasic person's ability to understand.

Speech sounds are not analyzed quickly enough for the patient to be able to hear a word accurately. The word "fork," for instance, may be heard as "pork" or "fort" or "sock." The problem is not one of deafness but of interpreting the nature of the speech sounds (vowels and consonants) as they arrive at the brain from the ear at the rate of about 14 per second.

The speech sounds themselves may be interpreted correctly, but the association between the sound of a word and what it means is lost or distorted. The word "fork," for instance, may be understood as "spoon"—the general idea is there, but the precise meaning is absent. In some instances, even the general idea appears to be lost, particularly for words that are used less frequently. In these cases the meaning of "house" would be retained, whereas the meaning of "edifice" might be lost.

Words themselves may be well understood, but the meaning that is conveyed by grammar—by how the words are strung together—may be lost or distorted. For instance, such a patient may understand a sentence such as "Bob wrote a check" but may not understand "Bob wrote Mary." In both cases, the patient would understand the meaning of the words "Bob," "wrote," "check," and "Mary," but word order no longer signifies. There is only one possible interpretation of the particular set of words of the first sentence: People write checks; checks do not write. However, correct interpretation of the second sentence depends on the knowledge that the first noun in most sentences (Bob, in this case) represents the person who does the action (writing, in this case), and that the second noun represents the person who receives the action. Other patients may remember the significance of word order in simple sentences such as this one but may not be able to understand complex sentences such as the passive (that is, they would infer from the sentence "The man was bitten by the dog" that the man, as the first noun of the sentence, had done the biting). Embedded sentences are also difficult for such patients to interpret. In this case, the sentence "The boy who hit the girl likes cheese" would be interpreted as "The boy hit the girl, and the girl likes cheese."

The patient may understand language better than it appears. Some patients may have paralysis or weakness of all of the muscles he would need in order to speak or gesture to indicate that he had understood. Other patients may have difficulty organizing or "programming" their motoric actions: They are "apraxic." Although they know what they want to do, they cannot seem to remember how to do it. They may try to comb their hair with their toothbrush, for instance, or try to put their arms through their pants legs when getting dressed. Such patients may make errors when following commands but not necessarily because they did not understand the command.

To summarize, what may appear as a problem in understanding the speech of others may or may not be a true language comprehension difficulty. Patients may not hear speech as speech; they may not be able to pay attention or concentrate; they may have a short-term memory loss. They may understand but not be able to talk, write, or gesture well enough to let the conversational partner know that they did indeed understand. However, all aphasic patients (those with damage in their dominant hemisphere, the left brain in most) have difficulty comprehending language. The difficulty varies according to the kind of aphasia and may range from a loss of part of the patient's vocabulary, to an impaired ability to interpret the sounds of words or relate words to their meaning, to an impaired ability to decipher the meaning conveyed by the grammar of a sentence. Naturally, the approach to rehabilitation varies with the underlying problem.

IMPAIRED EXPRESSION

Some patients are not able to express themselves adequately. As with the "comprehension" disorders, there is a broad range of possible difficulties in expression.

Nearly every stroke patient has some slurring of speech, particularly immediately after the stroke. One side of the face may droop, and there may be some weakness of the tongue, soft palate, and other muscles used for speech. Even though the patient may be saying perfectly normal sentences, the words are so "mushy" that the listener is hard put to understand. Weakness of the respiratory muscles or larynx (voice box) may make the voice weak and breathy, adding to the difficulty. This sort of "dysarthria" usually improves spontaneously over the course of a few days or weeks following a first stroke, leaving at most a mild slurring, particularly in patients whose strokes were in the right side of the brain.

Patients who have had more than one stroke may have an irreversible dysarthria. Both sides of the face may be weak, so that the patient cannot even close his mouth. The face is expressionless. The tongue and other muscles of the mouth can barely move. The voice may be harsh and "strangled" sounding. Attempts at speech are very difficult to understand, and because of the facial weakness the patient is unable to use facial expression to clarify his message. Many of these patients are considerably more intact intellectually and linguistically than they appear.

Some patients are able to speak but seldom try to do so. This lack of initiation is seen not just in speech but in activity of any kind. They simply sit and do nothing and say nothing, appearing to have little reaction, either physical or emotional, to anything in the environment. These patients are also unusually distractible, as described in the previous section, so that even if they have begun to say something they may stop in the middle of a sentence and behave as if they had forgotten what they were saying. The problem is not one of stubbornness, stupidity, or lack of motivation; nor is it one of depression apathy. It is caused by damage to that part of the brain (the front) which governs the planning and "switching on" of motoric actions.

The lack of activity described above could be called "inertia." Another aspect of inertia is the inability to stop an activity once started. This problem occurs in a great many stroke patients, some more than others. A response, once given correctly, keeps popping up in later conversation, inappropriately and virtually against the patient's will. One might ask the patient, for instance, what he would like to drink, and he might say "Coffee." Then, in response to subsequent questions, perhaps about the weather or the day's activities, he might continue to say "Coffee, no—coffee, no—coffee. . . ." This pattern is called "perseveration," and is usually beyond the control of the patient.

Some patients whose strokes were in the left side of the

brain are not able to program their speech muscles for speech production, similar to the apraxia involving the arms and legs described in the previous section. The two usually occur together, but "apraxia of speech" is occasionally seen in patients who otherwise have no apraxia involving their arms and legs. There are two basic types.

In one, the patient seems to have forgotten what to do with his mouth in order to produce speech sounds. He struggles to put his tongue in the right position, he stops and starts over again, distorting the speech sound with nearly every attempt. His speech is effortful and may be difficult to understand. In milder versions of this disorder the patients "trip over their own tongues" only occasionally; it happens particularly when they are thinking about what they are saying or when they are trying to imitate another's speech or to read aloud. At the other end of the spectrum, there are patients who are so severely apraxic they have actually forgotten how to turn on their voices. They can produce no volitional speech at all. However, they can cry out reflexively in pain or anger, and even the kindest and mildest mannered patient may be heard to swear, to the surprise of everyone who ever knew him. Some may have a stereotypical utterance which they repeat over and over again in any and all circumstances: "OK, OK, OK" or "home home home" or "doobie doobie doobie." Whatever these utterances are, they are not volitional speech and have no relation to what may be on the patient's mind. What is more, if such a patient is asked to produce any of these involuntary utterances of his own volition, he would probably be unable to do so.

In the other type of speech apraxia the individual speech sounds are relatively easily produced but are "out of alignment." Sounds or syllables may be borrowed from one word and repeated in another ("get a gorse" for "get a horse"), or they may be reversed ("het a gorse"). These difficulties with the sequencing of speech sounds are much like normal slips of the tongue in quality but occur much more frequently than they do in normal speech.

Many aphasic patients talk primarily in nouns, sometimes in nouns and verbs, leaving out all the connecting or descriptive words and sounding almost as if they were sending a telegram. It is "agrammatic" speech and is usually present in patients whose left-brain strokes left them with right-sided paralysis. These patients are called "Broca's aphasics," after the neurologist who first described such disorders. They may also have difficulty producing or sequencing speech sounds (the "apraxia" described above), particularly in the early days following the stroke, but the apraxia sometimes resolves, leaving the patient primarily agrammatic. Conversation must usually be carried on like a game of Twenty Questions, with the patient giving the general topic from his stock of nouns, and the listener guessing what the aphasic wants to say about the topic. For example, the patient might say "Mary . . . dishes . . . ," and it would be the listener's job to find out if Mary has done the dishes, broken the dishes, set the table, bought new dishes, etc. These patients appear to understand nearly everything that is said to them but usually have some difficulty understanding grammatically complex sentences and have particular difficulty understanding the meaning of "grammatical" words such as "before/after" and other prepositions. Nevertheless, they are usually relatively intact intellectually, are well aware of their communication problem, and are quite frustrated by their inability to express themselves adequately.

In sharp contrast to the effortful and telegraphic but relevant speech of the Broca's aphasic, the "Wernicke's aphasic" talks easily and endlessly, without appearing to say much. His speech contains a large proportion of descriptive and connective words, but his nouns may be limited to "thing" or other nonspecific terms. He rambles on, never really completing a sentence or conveying much, if any, information. Such patients usually have severe reduction in comprehension, in both interpreting speech sounds and associating sound with meaning, as described in the previous section. Their problems in understanding the meaning of words are reflected in their output. They may say "My ankle hurts" while showing by gesture that they have a headache. They may refer to a daughter as "sister," to a dinner knife as "spoon," or to a shoe as "sock." Some misnamings may be even further afield, showing a relation to the sound of the intended word rather than to its meaning: daughter as "potter," knife as "nice," shoe as "blue." In particularly severe cases the misnaming is so far afield that its relation to the intended word is not discernible to the listener: "ginter" for daughter, "plooth" for knife, "sooble" for shoe. Such patients are frequently unaware that their speech is incomprehensible to others and happily rattle on as if all were well with the world.

As described above, apraxic and aphasic patients (those with left-brain strokes) may have difficulty pronouncing words correctly, selecting the right words, or putting words together into complete and coherent sentences. Even the most severely impaired of these patients, however, are usually able to clarify their messages by their use of prosody—the stress and intonation, or musical quality, of speech. Even the patient who constantly uses only one word or phrase uses it with variations in loudness and pitch to express all kinds of emotion and to try to convey what is on his mind. Patients with right-brain strokes, on the other hand, frequently have considerable difficulty with prosodic or musical aspects of speech. Such patients may produce good speech in almost a monotone and thereby fail at conveying the emotional content of their messages. These individuals may also have difficulty guessing the emotional state of the person who is talking to them because of this difficulty in processing speech intonation.

Another important nonverbal means of communication is gesture. Obviously, an individual with only one functioning arm is somewhat handicapped in the use of gesture, but if the weakness or paralysis is the patient's biggest problem the gestures produced with the good arm should be of normal quality.

The gestures of aphasic patients are frequently of the same quality as their speech. That is, the Broca's type of aphasic—with hesitant, effortful, telegraphic speech—also has a limited repertoire of gestures that he uses sparingly but appropriately, whereas the Wernicke's type of aphasic—with rambling, incoherent speech—also may gesticulate a great deal without conveying much information. This rule holds true so long as the aphasia is not complicated by the type of apraxia mentioned in the section on comprehension (see above). Patients who cannot "program" the muscles of their hands and arms to do what they want them to are not likely to be able to convey much information by gesturing. Unfortunately, many of these patients are also aphasic, so the available channels for communicating are minimal.

Nearly all stroke patients, whether they are aphasic or not and whether their stroke was on the right or the left side of the brain, have some reduction in vocabulary. The amount of difficulty may be minimal in patients whose strokes were in the right side of the brain, but even the most mildly involved patient with left-brain involvement complains that he cannot remember names as well as before the stroke or has trouble working crossword puzzles. Such a patient might be embarrassed and surprised to find how few words he could come up with if asked to make a list of animals, foods, or items of clothing. The amount of difficulty that any given patient has generating word lists of this sort seems to be the best yardstick of the severity of the language impairment.

The vocabulary reduction is not necessarily uniform across all categories of words. Many patients have particular trouble remembering the names of body parts. Others have difficulty naming or recognizing the names of colors, even though they are not color blind. Such patients may also have trouble naming numbers (calling a "three" a "seven," for instance) even though they might be able to do arithmetic problems on paper; they may also have difficulty naming letters (calling the letter "c" "s," for instance) even though they might be able to read words. Nearly all have at least some trouble with "kinship terms" (words such as "husband," "mother," "uncle") and with the gender of personal pronouns, confusing "him" and "her," "he" and "she."

In general, the less frequently a word appears in our language, the more likely it is to disappear from the language of the aphasic patient. The person who might have used the word "edifice" before the stroke is now more likely to say "building," or "house," or "place," or "thing," depending on how severely his vocabulary is reduced.

To summarize, difficulty with verbal expression may vary from a purely physical problem with the clear pronunciation of speech related to weakness or incoordination of the muscles of the face and mouth, to impaired knowledge of how to create or sequence speech sounds, to an inability to produce grammatically complete sentences, to a reduced ability to relay information in a coherent fashion. Expression of emotion may also be impaired by an inability to adjust the "musical" aspects of speech: stress and intonation. Gestural expression may also be impaired by weakness or apraxia of the upper limbs, and the quality of gestures probably mirrors the quality of the speech of aphasic patients. No matter what the basic problem, it is accompanied by some reduction in vocabulary. As with the comprehension problems, the underlying problem and its severity influence the design of the rehabilitation program.

IMPAIRED ABILITY TO READ OR WRITE

Some patients cannot read or write as well as before the stroke. As with the other deficits, this mode of communication may be impaired in a variety of ways.

Patients who are dysarthric, as described in the previous section, may have some physical difficulty moving a pencil across a page if their dominant hand is weak or paralyzed. If there is no accompanying language disturbance (reduced initiation, perseveration, apraxia, aphasia), such individuals may easily learn to write with their nondominant hand. If vision has not been impaired by the stroke, reading is probably not a problem.

Those patients who do not initiate speech and those who perseverate, as described in the previous section, are quite likely to show the same behavioral patterns when requested to write. Their reading and writing may, in addition, be impaired in one of the manners described elsewhere in this chapter.

In general, most of us write about the same way we talk, and we do not understand an unfamiliar word in print any better than we would if we heard it. It stands to reason, then, that the individual whose language system has been impaired by a left-brain stroke is no better at reading and writing than he is at verbal communication. This statement is the case in the average, uncomplicated aphasia or apraxia of speech as described in the foregoing sections. However, there are exceptions to every rule, including this one, and there are occasional cases of reading and/or writing disturbances that seem much more severe than the verbal language disturbance.

Some patients with left-brain strokes have lost the connection between what a word looks like on the printed page and what it sounds like. Such a patient may know the alphabet and be able to name letters when he sees them but has forgotten how they sound in speech and therefore is not able to read by "sounding out" words. Some words are recognized and understood visually, as a "gestalt" or whole, even though the patient cannot remember how to say the word. He may look at the word "jacket" and say "coat," for instance, or wordlessly pretend to put on a jacket, showing that he understood the general meaning of the word. There may be many words, however, that the patient does not recognize visually, and in these cases his inability to "sound out" leaves him hopelessly incapable of deciphering them. This condition has been referred to as "deep dyslexia." Depending on the severity of the disorder, the patient may be able to understand written messages better than he can read them aloud because he makes some educated guesses based on whatever words he is able to recognize.

"Surface dyslexia" is almost a negative image of the deep dyslexia described above. In this disorder, the patient does not visually recognize any words at all, but he does remember how to "sound out" words letter by letter. He can thus read aloud, and once he hears himself say the word he understands what it is. It is, of course, a laborious method of reading at best and is complicated by the fact that English spelling has so many irregularities. A patient with this disorder, for instance, might read the word "dough" as "duff" (as in "enough") and thus would not understand it, as his visual recognition of words has been lost. Overall, therefore, this sort of patient probably does not understand written language as well as the deep dyslexic, even though he is better able to read aloud.

Many patients with right-brain strokes tend to "neglect" the left side of space. These individuals have lost their vision to the left, but the neglect goes far beyond a simple visual impairment. Such patients may not recognize their left arm or leg as their own; they may ignore the food on the left side of their plate; they may comb their hair only on the right side; and they may not even turn their head or eyes to the left when they hear something from that direction. There may be some neglect of the right side of space in patients with left-brain strokes, but it usually resolves within a few days or weeks, even though the right-sided visual loss remains. Left side neglect frequently affects reading and writing, in that the patients tend to act as if the left side of the page were not there. If asked to read aloud, they may read from the middle to the end of the line, drop down a line and begin again at the middle of the next line. They have little or no difficulty deciphering the individual words, but they obviously have difficulty deciphering the message if they are reading only half of each line. Similarly, when attempting to write, these patients usually start at the middle of the page and continue writing to the very edge of the page, if not off it and onto the table. The line of writing usually slopes downward, and as the patient runs out of space he may think nothing of writing one word on top of the previous one, rather than turning the page. The handwriting may be considerably less legible than before the stroke, even though the patient is writing with the unaffected, dominant right hand. This pattern is related to the patient's difficulty in dealing with the visual-spatial domain; drawing may be similarly impaired.

Occasionally, patients with left-brain strokes also have difficulty with writing that goes beyond the mere problem of having to use the nondominant hand (left, in most cases). When they pick up the pencil to write or draw, they may make random marks on the page that look like nothing at all, and they can no more draw than they can write. This situation is, in a sense, an "apraxia of writing." These patients, as those with right-brain strokes described above, may also have difficulty dressing and solving arithmetic problems, both of which also require manipulating things in space: arranging clothing on the body in one case, aligning numbers on a page in the other.

In summary, reading and writing are probably impaired to some degree in anyone who has had a stroke. The severity and underlying cause of the problem vary according to the side of the brain involved and to the location of the stroke within that side of the brain. In some cases the functional result is trivial, whereas in others it is devastating. Some disorders are easily overcome, and others are irreversible. Again, the nature and severity of the disorder influence the approach to rehabilitation.

THE PATIENT—A "CHANGED PERSON"

The patient does not seem to be the "same person" as before the stroke. To some degree, every stroke patient seems

to have become "different." Disruption of normal communication channels naturally alters the relation of the patient to
his family and friends, but some emotional and intellectual
factors have an even greater influence on the patient's behavior and on the perception of the patient by those who know
him.

Emotionally, the patient is frequently seen as having become a "caricature" of his former self: All his good qualities
are exaggerated, as are all his bad qualities. His patience and
self-control may be lost. There may be large, unexpected
mood swings. The patient may be anxious and dependent one
moment and angry and resentful the next. One of the most
striking emotional changes is the easy crying of the stroke
patient, often for no apparent reason. Other patients seem to
have almost no emotion at all and can discuss the most tragic
of topics as if they were talking about a picnic in the park.
This does not necessarily mean that the patient does not truly
have any emotions. It is sometimes difficult to tell the difference between true lack of emotion and the inability to put
"music" in one's speech as discussed in the section on expressive language (see above). Whatever the problem, most
patients are aware of and bothered by these new behaviors,
this new loss of inhibition. It is generally beyond the control
of the patient and the direct result of the damage done to the
brain by the stroke.

Any damage to the brain serious enough to have caused
other symptoms probably has also caused some reduction of
intellect. The important thing to remember about the communication disorders (aphasia, apraxia of speech, dysarthria)
is that the language or speech dysfunction is usually much
more severe than the intellectual dysfunction. Unfortunately,
we humans tend to judge one another by the way we talk, and
a person who has difficulty talking "normally" is usually considered to be intellectually inferior. In most instances, communicatively impaired patients can think and have concepts

in their heads that they are unable to express adequately. Tragically, however, there are patients, particularly those with massive strokes or those who have had a series of smaller strokes, who may have truly lost a great deal of their ability to think or who may have lost entire concepts, not merely the words with which to express those concepts. Such an individual, for instance, may not only be unable to name a cup when it is placed in his hand but also may not know what to do with it: He may try to use it as a razor or a floor mop, for instance. Such a patient, after being taught that pottery mugs, large china teacups, and smaller demitasse cups are all called "cup," might be surprised to learn that a similarly shaped tin cup could also be called "cup." This is obviously a much more severe disorder than the inability to recall the name of that object on the saucer or the misnaming of it as a "pup" (similar in sound) or a "dish" (similar in function), as would happen in aphasia. Such reductions in thought, however, are not necessarily accompanied by a reduction in the patient's sense of self.

All of these disorders are most severe during the first weeks or months, with some spontaneous recovery expected in nearly all patients. Rehabilitation may enhance the natural course of recovery and may indeed continue to improve the patient's communicative functioning after spontaneous recovery has ceased. It is important to remember, however, that few if any communicatively impaired individuals will ever regain their prior facility with the language, and the major functions of speech therapy are first to see to it that the patient makes maximum use of his remaining language capacity and then to assist the patient and the patient's family in accepting and coping with the disorder. An understanding of the natural course or evolution of the communication disorders following stroke may prepare the reader to consider the roles of the speech/language pathologist, the patient, and the family in rehabilitation.

NATURAL COURSE OF COMMUNICATION DISORDERS FOLLOWING STROKE

When speech or language disorders occur following stroke, they are at their worst during the first few days, after which there is almost always some improvement. No one ever gets worse unless there has been an intervening medical complication, such as another stroke.

Unlike the muscles of the face, arms, and legs, the oral muscles (tongue, soft palate, pharynx, larynx) are capable of receiving commands from both sides of the brain. Therefore if the problem is purely one of dysarthria (the "slurring" of speech as a result of muscle weakness), it should improve dramatically within a few weeks, as the weakened muscles begin to accept commands from the undamaged side of the brain. The drooping mouth is likely to remain, leaving some difficulty in the production of sounds made with the lips (p, b, m). These statements apply only to first strokes. Additional strokes, particularly on the other side of the brain, would seriously reduce the chances for recovery of speech.

With or without therapy, the maximum improvement in the aphasic patient (including the apraxic patient) is seen during about the first month. The rate of natural recovery remains rapid for the next 2 months or so; it then slows down and finally ceases by the sixth to twelfth month following the stroke. With speech therapy, however, some aphasic patients have been reported to show improvement even years after their strokes.

Although nearly every aphasic patient improves (with or without therapy), few recover completely. There is often dramatic improvement during the first days or weeks, but the person who is still aphasic by the time he or she is medically stable and ready for discharge from the hospital is likely to remain aphasic to some extent, despite continued improvement after discharge. At best, there is residual difficulty in word retrieval (naming). At worst, the improvement is so slight, particularly in the profoundly impaired, that it has little effect on the patient's functional ability to communicate. As a rule of thumb, we could say that the amount of impairment at about a month following onset is a good predictor of the amount of natural recovery to be expected: the more severe the aphasia at 1 month, the less recovery to be expected by 6 months.

Other factors also may affect recovery from aphasia. Left-handed individuals as a rule recover better than right-handed individuals, probably because language competence is less lateralized (less restricted to the left side of the brain) in left-handers, and so there is more language available in the undamaged areas of the brain. Younger people (under 60 years old) are sometimes reported to recover better than older people, but younger people also often have less serious forms of aphasia to start with, so the recovery is probably related more to severity than to age.

The type of stroke incurred may influence recovery from aphasia. Individuals with nonocclusive infarctions (diminished blood flow without evidence of arterial blockage) are more likely to improve than those with arterial blockage. Patients with brain hemorrhages are frequently more severely aphasic to begin with and often do not improve as well as patients with brain infarctions. As with the dysarthrias, massive strokes, multiple strokes, and particularly strokes in both sides of the brain make the outlook for recovery from aphasia gloomy.

In general, comprehension seems to improve more than the fluency of expressive language. The person who has to struggle to get words out will probably have that sort of difficulty for the rest of his life, at least to some extent, but his ability to follow what is being said to him may well improve.

Of course, there are exceptions to every rule. No two people are alike; no two brains are alike; no two aphasias are alike. Some patients seem to improve against all odds; others surprise everyone by not living up to their potential. Factors such as personality, motivation, education, intelligence, family support, general health, and coexisting medical complications influence the patient's recovery.

During the period of natural recovery and beyond, the patient and the family must learn to adjust, to compensate, to cope. The goal of rehabilitation is to maximize the patient's ability to communicate, given the specific nature of his language loss. Some may be able to reach this goal on their own. Most find the help of a speech/language pathologist a necessary part of the rehabilitation process. What are the roles of the therapist, the family, and the patient in rehabilitation?

Role of the Speech/Language Pathologist

The inability to make oneself understood is a rather frightening experience. In the early days following onset of the stroke, both the patient and family must make some major adjustments to a new situation. Direct therapy at this point is probably not a good idea, but in many hospitals the speech/language pathologist is called on to assess the patient and advise the medical team on how best to communicate with the patient. The therapist can determine if the patient would be able to use a nonverbal means of communication; he also provides whatever aids may be appropriate and trains the patient, family, and medical staff in their use. He can recognize what communication channels are the least impaired and reinforce the patient's efforts to use them, paving the way for subsequent therapy. As it turns out, the speech/language pathologist frequently becomes the intermediary between the family and the physician and other hospital personnel, making sure that the family understands the diagnosis and prognosis as given by the physician, as well as making sure that the medical team is aware of the family's particular concerns.

Once the patient has stabilized and is ready to take part in the rehabilitation process, the first duty of the clinician (speech/language pathologist) is to thoroughly assess the patient's communicative strengths and weaknesses.

Tests for dysarthria allow the clinician to judge the manner in which speech sounds are produced and to compare speech patterns to the changes that have taken place in the patient's speech musculature. An assessment is done, if necessary, of changes that can be made in the environment or in the patient's posture that could improve his ability to make himself understood in the short run. Therapy goals for the long run are based on what the clinician learns about the patient from testing and on what the clinician knows to be the pattern of progression of the patient's particular disorder.

As the reader can recall, aphasia and apraxia are complex disorders, with many potential problems underlying any given superficial symptom. Intelligent therapy planning depends on thorough testing of the aphasic/apraxic patient. Ideally, the speech/language pathologist, using one or more of a number of comprehensive language tests, assesses the following: (a) The patient's production of conversational speech, looking for the amount of speech produced, the ease with which it is produced, the length and type of sentences used, and the amount of information conveyed; (b) the patient's comprehension of words, sentences, and paragraphs under a variety of conditions; (c) the patient's naming ability under a variety of conditions; (d) the patient's ability to imitate words, phrases, and sentences; (e) the patient's ability to read aloud and to understand what is read; (f) the patient's physical ability to draw and write, as well as the content or quality of his drawing and writing; (g) the patient's ability to produce gestures; (h) the patient's ability to do arithmetic problems; (i) the patient's orientation, knowledge, and general ability to respond in the clinical situation.

All of these functions are assessed in a standardized fashion so the results can be compared with those of a large group of other aphasic individuals. The assessment allows the clinician to determine the kind of disorder he is dealing with, how severe it is, and what the relative strengths and weaknesses of the patient are. All items on a good standardized aphasia test are carefully chosen to minimize the effects of education. These tests are not intelligence tests but are designed to uncover language changes that are the direct result of the stroke.

Given all the test results, the clinician determines whether therapy would be beneficial for the patient, and if so what type of therapy is appropriate. As an example, suppose that a patient has difficulty naming things. The reasons for this difficulty have been uncovered by the language testing, and the clinician now steps in and works on the underlying problem.

It may be that the patient cannot name because he cannot adequately control his speech muscles. The clinician would probably begin by retraining muscle control for simple facial and oral movements before beginning to work on isolated sounds, then on simple words, then on longer and longer utterances. If the problem is particularly severe, the clinician will probably try to provide an appropriate alternative means of communication until the patient's verbal channel can take over. If the patient's writing is relatively intact, writing is encouraged. If the patient cannot write, it is highly unlikely that he can use an alphabet board. If the patient can produce gestures adequately, a gestural system may be introduced. If the patient cannot write or gesture, which he probably is not able to do, but can read simple words and phrases, a phrase board is designed with messages the patient can point to. If the patient's reading is also poor, a picture board may be designed.

It may be that the naming disorder is one of retrieval: the "tip-of-the-tongue" phenomenon. Sometimes the connection between a word and the object or action or attribute to which that word refers (the "referent") has been disrupted. The word itself and the concept of the referent are both there in the patient's mind, but the word just cannot be brought to mind without some sort of cueing. It is the sort of naming problem that confronts all of us from time to time; it is simply more frequent in aphasia. Testing would have revealed the type of cueing that may be most helpful to the patient for retrieving the desired word. Sometimes hearing the first sound or syllable of the word helps. In other cases, seeing the first few letters of the word helps. Sometimes hearing a rhyming word may help. Whatever the type of cueing the individual patient responds to best, the clinician begins by providing the maximum amount necessary for the individual patient—no more and no less than required to assist in retrieval of the desired word. Step by step the clinician then withdraws cueing, training the patient in one way or another to cue himself.

It may be that the naming disorder is more serious than the retrieval problem described above. Sometimes the concept of the referent is diminished in scope. That is, the word does not mean quite as much to the patient as it had before. Consider the meaning of the word "apple," for instance. Its full meaning includes what an apple looks like (size, shape, color), what it smells and tastes like, what it feels like (weight and shape and smoothness in the hand, crunchiness in the mouth), and even what it sounds like when being bitten into and chewed. Each of these sensations has entered the brain through different channels and may therefore have been stored in different areas of the brain. There are patients who, when confronted with an apple, for instance, genuinely do not know what it is by simply looking at it but who instantly recognize it when it is placed in their hands or when they take a bite of it. This type of partial recognition is presumably because the area of the brain that stored visual memories of apples has been damaged by the stroke, but the areas that stored other types of memories of apples are still intact. Such a patient might not be able to tell you what an apple looks like but would probably be able to tell you that it is good to eat. Other patients might not recognize an apple by its feel if they are blindfolded or in a dark room; but they will recognize it when they look at it. This loss of knowledge about objects has the technical name "agnosia." In these instances, it is doubtful that the lost bits of knowledge about apples (and other referents, which are affected in a similar fashion) can be replaced. The patient needs to learn to cope with his diminished knowledge, relying on what he does know about things.

There are more severe "naming" disorders of this general nature, in which the concept of a referent is diminished in more than one modality. If an individual does not recognize an apple when he looks at it, when he holds it in his hand, or when he tastes it, he has truly lost the idea of an apple. This is obviously much more serious than forgetting the name of an apple. If these patients improve at all, they probably do so in response to daily contact with family members in a familiar environment and not from occasional visits to a speech clinic.

With some aphasic naming disorders, the concept of "apple" (for instance) may be diminished to a minimal extent, but the major problem is that access to the word "apple" is blocked through one or another channel, similar to the "tip-of-the-tongue" phenomenon described earlier. For instance, such a patient may not be able to name an apple when looking at it or even when visualizing it in his "mind's eye." However, he is most likely to say "Oh, what's the name of that thing!" The previously described agnosic individual, on the other hand, would say "I don't know what that is," and the patient with the "tip-of-the-tongue" problem might say "Oh yes, that's a happer, a packle, an a-. . . ." The aphasic patient who cannot name the apple when looking at it may be able to remember the word for it if he puts the apple in his hand or bites into it.

Although all these individuals appear to have the same difficulty naming objects, the underlying disorders are different. An accurate evaluation of the patient is essential because some disorders are more amenable to treatment than others. The person whose knowledge is relatively intact but who has difficulty retrieving words may, for instance, be trained to cue himself through his intact channels. If access to the word through the visual channel is blocked, the patient can be trained to imagine an object's feel, taste, or function, for example. This method may not work, however, for the patient whose general knowledge has been diminished. Only careful testing can determine the underlying problem.

Just as there may be more than one reason for a person's trouble with naming, there may be more than one reason for problems with putting words together into sentences, understanding speech, reading and understanding written material, and writing. As with the naming disorders, it is important to have a professional speech/language pathologist evaluate the situation, determine whether therapy would be beneficial, and, if so, design a program specifically for the individual. This program will carry the patient through a series of steps, beginning at his current level and gradually increasing in difficulty until he reaches his potential. When well designed, it allows the patient to concentrate on only one thing at a time. Without the guidance of a speech/language pathologist, attempts at therapy by family members or volunteers may do more harm than good, frustrating both the patient and the person who is trying to help. Problems may develop because the "homemade" program is attacking the wrong underlying disorder, because it is asking more of the patient than he is currently capable of, or because it is demanding attention to more than one thing at a time.

The professionally designed program may be carried out by the clinician and/or family members and may include any or all of the following: (a) restoration of as much speech and language function as the patient is capable of achieving; (b) compensation for lost function through intact speech or language channels; (c) substitution of nonverbal methods of communication. The latter ranges from simple communication boards with pictures to which the patient may point to computerized environmental control systems with speech synthesizers, depending on the patient's needs and capabilities. No matter what the goals of rehabilitation, the process requires a lot of time and effort on the part of the patient and clinician, as well as the family.

As in the acute stage, the speech/language pathologist is frequently called on during the rehabilitative stage to provide counseling to the patient and the family. It sometimes takes a while for the long-term implications of the speech or language impairment to "soak in" and for the patient and those close to him to accept the fact that communication will probably never return to its previous, normal state, even with therapy. However, while helping the patient to attain his maximum potential communicative abilities, the clinician also helps the patient and those around him to accept and adjust to the new circumstances, to recognize the difference between impaired communication and impaired reason, to face up to their feelings about themselves and each other in these new circumstances, and to resume as normal a personal relationship as may have existed before the stroke.

The final step toward independence is often the most difficult but is certainly the most important: terminating therapy as soon as further progress becomes improbable. It is difficult because all concerned hope that continued therapy will continue to improve the patient's communication. It is important to recognize this point because false hope delays final acceptance of and adjustment to the disability. Life does go on, and with adequate therapy and counseling both patient and family can be confident that it is going on as well as could possibly be expected.

Role of the Patient and Family

Rehabilitation is possible only if the therapist, the patient, and the patient's family agree that there is a problem worthy of rehabilitation, that the patient would be capable of responding significantly to therapy, and that there is adequate time to devote to the process of rehabilitation. Note that all three parties must agree.

If the patient, his family, or both consider the communication disorder significant enough to warrant rehabilitation, it may be their responsibility to insist on therapy, even though the clinician may disagree. In such cases a few sessions of "trial" or "diagnostic" therapy may serve either to convince the clinician that the problem is amenable to treatment or to convince the patient and family that it is not. In either case, the ultimate outcome is satisfaction that everything possible has been done for the patient's communication problem.

Even if everyone should agree that there is a problem that could be treated, successful rehabilitation requires considerable time and effort on the parts of all concerned. The patient and his family must be prepared to spend a portion of every day practicing tasks prescribed by the clinician. Time spent with the therapist, whether in the clinic or at home, must be in productive therapy or focused counseling; it must not be looked on as social visits or "baby-sitting." Not only must the patient and family dedicate a measurable portion of their time to therapy tasks, the patient must also have the stamina and determination to continue participation in an effort that is truly effort. Any changes made in the patient's ability to communicate are made despite a damaged nervous system that is no longer capable of handling communication in a "normal" fashion. There may come a time when the patient decides that further effort is not worth it. That is the patient's decision, and it should be respected by the clinician and the family. Again, the ultimate outcome is satisfaction that everything possible has been done for the patient's communication problem. The next step is getting on with life within the context of the patient's disability.

GUIDELINES FOR COMMUNICATING WITH THE COMMUNICATIVELY HANDICAPPED PATIENT

As the reader must have accepted by now, patients differ widely in their communicative disorders and in the basic problems underlying these disorders. Therefore any "cookbook" type of recommendations, including the ones provided below, are to be taken with a grain of salt. The speech/language pathologist who evaluates the patient, regardless of whether therapy is recommended, provides specific guidelines for communication, given the patient's specific disability. The following ideas, however, apply in most situations.

1. Patients who have the most difficulty making themselves understood often (but not always) have the least difficulty understanding what others say to them. Do not make assumptions about the patient's language comprehension or about his "mind" on the basis of the way he talks.

2. Patients who have difficulty producing and/or understanding speech as the result of a stroke have not suddenly become deaf. There is no need to shout. Furthermore, the best assumption is that even the most severely impaired patient may be able to understand what you are saying, even in a whisper, so consider his feelings before talking about him in his presence.

3. Patients who have difficulty producing and/or understanding speech as the result of a stroke have not suddenly become babies or simpletons. They would thank you for not addressing them with baby talk or talking down to them in any fashion. They appreciate being included in family discussions and social gatherings as the adults that they are, and they want to participate in any family decisions that are made. They resent having others make decisions for them, just as they resent having others talk for them when, given a little time and effort, they may have been able to get the message across themselves.

4. Patients whose communication difficulties seem worse on some days than on others, or at some times of the day than at others, cannot help it. They are already frustrated by the problems they have communicating their thoughts to others. They become further frustrated if you demand something of

them of which they are incapable at the moment, even though they might have been capable of it only a few moments ago. Pointing out their inconsistencies at such a time does not help them overcome the immediate problem. Always remember that they are doing the best they can.

5. Patients are usually aware of their problems and the seriousness of them. Do not belittle or insult them by well-intentioned remarks such as "Everything is going to be all right." Let the patient know that you recognize how difficult it is for him to communicate. Express your admiration of his attempts at communication, and do not demand more than he is capable of giving. If the patient is so impaired that he is unable to do so himself, express his anger and frustration for him. This situation is the only one in which it may be necessary to talk "for" the patient, and you may find that it not only relieves some of the patient's frustration but some of your own as well, as the two of you face the problem head-on, honestly and openly. Remember also that it is all right to cry.

In addition to the above, the following guidelines may help communication with aphasic patients who are having particular difficulty understanding speech: Slow down just a little to give the patient's brain a little more time to make sense of your message. Do not slow down too much, or the patient may have trouble remembering the first part of your message by the time you get to the end of it. Try to talk in short and simple but complete, natural sentences. Do not talk too much: Say what needs to be said and then quit. If the patient seems confused by what you said, try saying it another way. Use facial expression and body language to supplement and clarify your message. Remember that he probably cannot understand writing or a formal gestural language (such as sign language) any better than he does speech. Do not attempt these types of communication unless specifically recommended by the therapist. Turn off the radio or television and keep other competing noise to a minimum when trying to talk to the patient.

If there are several people around, see to it that only one person speaks at a time. Remember: the patient is neither deaf nor stupid nor a child.

The following suggestions may make life a little easier for the patients who are having particular difficulty expressing themselves. Patients who are dysarthric—whose problems are exclusively with the physical production of speech and not with the formulation of language—may need to remind themselves to slow down in order to give their speech muscles time to make the moves necessary for clearer speech production. They may find that they can make themselves understood better if they say one word at a time. They may be able to write, if their visual system and their writing hand have not been impaired by the stroke. Further suggestions from the patient's speech/language pathologist are based on the patient's specific disorder.

Whether he is aphasic, apraxic, or dysarthric, if you cannot understand what the patient is saying, try asking questions he can answer with a simple "yes" or "no." If the patient says "yes" to everything, it is not necessarily because he does not understand the questions, nor is it necessarily because he really means "yes." He may be perseverating. In such cases, a simple head nod or head shake may work better, or you may need to rely on the patient's facial expression to tell when he means "yes" and when he means "no." This method of yes/no questioning requires some sensitivity to the patient and his concerns—and a great deal of patience. Just as in a game of Twenty Questions, you first try to discover the general topic and then narrow it down until you are satisfied that you have understood what was on the patient's mind. If the patient, for instance, appears to be worried about something and is struggling to talk to you, you might proceed as follows: "Are you worried about the kids? . . . about the garden? . . . about money?" Suppose the patient says "no" (or shakes his head) to the first two, and indicates that the last is the topic of concern. Your next job would be to list the money concerns that might be troubling the patient: "Is it the mortgage payments? . . . The hospital bills? . . . The car insurance?" Once the narrowed topic has been discovered, you would continue to ask yes/no questions until the patient, through your help, has been able to communicate his concerns. The effectiveness of this method of communication depends on your understanding of the patient and the things he is most likely to want to talk about, as well as the patient's comprehension of your speech. Remember the guidelines for talking to the aphasic patient with comprehension problems.

If the patient gets "stuck" on a word and keeps repeating it (perseverating) regardless of what he is trying to say, it is sometimes the best course of action to stop the conversation and resume it a little later. This gives the patient the time to "erase the board," and you may find that communication is then easier for a time. This method again requires a great deal of patience and understanding on the part of the listener.

Remember that the aphasic patient is unlikely to be able to write, spell, or gesture any better than he can speak. Do not try to make him use one of these other language channels unless specifically recommended by the speech/language pathologist after a thorough evaluation of his abilities.

As stated before, always remember that despite the speech or language disability, the patient has remained an adult, with adult feelings and concerns. To assume otherwise is unfair to him and to you.

SOURCES OF THERAPY AND OTHER SUPPORT SERVICES

Most hospitals have speech/language pathologists on their staffs. These clinicians provide evaluation and treatment services in the hospital after they receive a consultation request from the patient's physician. Such services are covered by Medicare but may not be covered by private health insurance plans. When in doubt, check the insurance policy or with the insurance agent.

Outpatient speech/language therapy can be reimbursed only if it has been prescribed by a physician. As of this writing, Medicare, Part A, pays 100% of the costs of speech/language therapy in a Medicare-sponsored skilled nursing home or through a Home Health Agency, so long as certain requirements are met. Therapy must be considered reasonable and necessary, must require the skill of a trained professional, and must continue to produce progress. Medicare, Part B, covers speech/language therapy through a rehabilitation agency in the patient's home, a private clinic, or any nursing home, regardless of whether it is Medicare-sponsored, so long as the above requirements are met. As with hospital treatment, some insurance policies cover outpatient speech/language therapy, and some do not. Even though the patient may not be eligible for reimbursement for therapy, the services of a certified therapist may be desirable.

How does one go about finding a speech/language pathologist? The physician or the local Easter Seal Society or Heart Association may be able to recommend one. Most cities have rehabilitation agencies staffed with speech/language pathologists who are nationally certified and/or state licensed. If the patient lives in a community with a university that has a communication disorders or speech/language pathology department, therapy may be done at reduced rates, as it is provided by student therapists in training under the direct supervision of certified speech/language pathologists. If the patient is a veteran, he may be eligible for treatment free of charge at the local Veterans Administration Hospital. If none of these options is available, contact the American Speech–Language–Hearing Association, 10801 Rockville Pike, Rockville, Maryland 20852 and ask for a list of speech/language pathologists in the area. This organization certifies and maintains records on speech/language pathologists throughout the United States.

Patients with communication disorders often find it difficult to maintain an adequate social life and so feel left out and "different" in their previous social group. Many communities have a Stroke Club, sponsored by a local hospital or university or by the local chapter of the American Heart Association or some other service agency. Even if individual therapy is not recommended or desired, participation in such a club or group activity is often beneficial, as the patient learns that he is not alone with his handicap and he acquires more self-confidence in communicating in an understanding environment. Again, it is important to search out such groups by contacting the same organizations and agencies noted above.

A newsletter by and for aphasic patients, *A Stroke of Luck,* is published quarterly and can be ordered from Mrs. Helen Wulf (herself an aphasic) at 9305 Waterview Road, Dallas, Texas 75218. In it patients describe their unique problems, ask questions, and provide moral support for one another across the United States. A few biographical and autobiographical accounts of recovery from aphasia are included in the references at the end of this chapter.

Moral support is probably the most important part of rehabilitating patients with language and speech problems following stroke. That support must be provided by all the people who care for the patient: physician, therapists, fellow patients, family, friends. Perhaps some of the guidelines in this chapter can remind all concerned of the basic humanity of the patient, no matter how severely impaired his communication may be. In return for this support—and often despite the lack of it— the patient gives his utmost, first to become the best communicator he can and then to contribute his best to normal family, social, and civic relationships.

REFERENCES

1. Boone, D. (1983): *An Adult Has Aphasia.* Interstate Printers & Publishers, Danville, Illinois.
2. Buck, M. (1968): *Dysphasia: Professional Guidance for Family and Patient.* Prentice-Hall, Englewood Cliffs, New Jersey.

3. DeMille, A. (1981): *Reprieve: A Memoire*. Doubleday, Garden City, New York.
4. Farrell, B. (1969): *Pat and Roald*. Random House, New York.
5. Luria, A. R. (1972): *The Man with a Shattered World*. Basic Books, New York.
6. Moss, C. (1972): *Recovery with Aphasia: The Aftermath of My Stroke*. University of Illinois Press, Urbana.
7. Wulf, H. (1974): *Aphasia: My World Alone*. Wayne State University Press, Detroit.

12

Spatial–Perceptual Deficits

J. Stanwood Till

The stroke patient with right-brain damage often has difficulty with the ability to judge distance, size, position, and speed, as well as how individual parts of an object relate to the whole. Such difficulties are termed spatial–perceptual deficits. Often a patient with right-brain damage has good speech and is able to articulate plans so well that the family tends to believe him and is therefore easily fooled about his true abilities. These patients may have trouble reading newspapers or adding columns of figures, not because they lack the ability to read or add but because they lose their place while trying to perform either of these tasks. They may miss buttons when buttoning their shirts, or they may confuse the inside and outside of the clothes they wear. Those who are helping to take care of right-brain stroke victims often confuse this inability caused by spatial–perceptual deficits with being uncooperative, unmotivated, recalcitrant, or confused.

Those with left-brain damage (right-sided weakness) may be quite slow and cautious, and tend not to take on even tasks that are equal to their mental and physical abilities. On the other hand, patients with right-brain damage (that is, a patient with left-sided weakness) may behave in a manner that promotes overestimation of their actual abilities. This patient tends to be impulsive and often attempts things too quickly. He may try to walk across a room without putting his brace

159

on or, what is even more dangerous, may attempt to drive a car without being aware of the extent of his deficit.

The patient with damage to the right side of his brain also needs a great deal of feedback when he is attempting to learn a new task. He needs to be encouraged to slow down and to check each step carefully before he goes on to the next. Having the patient talk his way through physical tasks is usually quite useful and makes the task easier to perform. It is important for persons involved in the care of these patients to try to make most of their feedback of a positive nature rather than nagging and being overly critical, which tend to discourage any further effort on the part of the patient.

Patients with spatial–perceptual deficits may have difficulty understanding visual clues they receive from the environment. Often a highly involved, intricate environment with loud, complicated geometric wallpaper causes a great deal of spatial confusion for them. It is important to have a well-lit room with a limited number of objects and a relatively slow, uncongested traffic pattern.

NEGLECT

Many patients who have had a major stroke have a loss of half of their visual field, usually on the same side as the weak body parts; that is, patients with right-sided weakness tend to have a right field cut, whereas those with left-sided weakness have a left field cut. Field cuts can be imagined as trying to look out at the world through a pair of glasses with black tape over half of each lens. The only way to truly see the total environment is to turn the head. Usually stroke patients learn to compensate for the visual field loss by turning their eyes or their head. In some cases, however, the stroke patient does not seem to learn to compensate for the visual field loss and, instead, seems to neglect the portion of the visual field he cannot perceive.

In general, individuals with left-sided weakness seem to

have more problems with neglect than those with right-sided weakness. For example, the individual with left-sided weakness may not recognize his own arm and leg as being part of his body. Often this patient awakens in the middle of the night wondering who is in bed with him.

Dealing with patients with neglect requires special considerations. It is important to address the patient from his unimpaired side and to situate him in a room so that the unimpaired side as well as unimpaired visual field is toward the main area of activity, usually toward the door to the room. Positioning the patient so that the impaired side is facing the room and the unimpaired side is facing a wall makes him feel completely isolated because he cannot see what is going on in the room, seeing only the wall. Occasionally, patients with neglect not only ignore the visual field on the side of their weakness but often actually divide the things they see right at the midline and seem to accept this limitation as the way things are. An example is the patient who is eating dinner but eats food only on the right side of the plate, ignoring all the food on the left side until the plate is rotated 180 degrees.

Patients with neglect are often easily confused when traveling. If the patient is wheeled down a hallway with the nonneglect side facing one side of the corridor, on the way back the nonneglect visual field faces the opposite side of the corridor. Therefore from the standpoint of the patient, he is seeing a completely different hallway. It often helps to point out the various landmarks on the right and left sides, thereby familiarizing the patient with the overall scene.

It is helpful to give the patient with neglect as much feedback as possible about his neglected limbs. Tying a bell or a ribbon around a neglected limb often calls a patient's attention to the fact that it is his own arm or leg. Again, it is important not to nag the patient about the impairment but, rather, to make constructive comments, thereby helping him deal with his impairment.

13

Bladder and Bowel Problems

Nancy Crater

If there is damage to the higher centers of the brain from a stroke voluntary control of the urinary bladder may be affected, leading to bladder incontinence (lack of control) or retention of urine. On the other hand, bowel problems usually are seen as the side effect or result of the other complaints of stroke and not of the brain damage itself. Bladder and bowel problems can be both frustrating and embarrassing to the individual and his family. Management begins as soon as the problem is recognized; it is aimed at reestablishing a normal pattern.

BLADDER PROBLEMS

Bladder problems are usually due to a breakdown in the transmission of messages between the brain and the bladder. The two most common bladder problems after a stroke are (a) the inability to pass urine from the bladder, referred to as urinary retention; and (b) the inability to control the passage of urine from the bladder, or urinary incontinence. The latter is more common.

The above problems are symptoms and thus do not reveal the whole picture. When one of these problems persists, a kidney and bladder evaluation should be performed. This workup, along with a complete prestroke urinary history, helps determine if the problem is due to the stroke or to another disorder (tumor, infection, etc.).

Treatment of Urinary Problems

During the acute stage a small catheter may be inserted into the bladder to facilitate removal of urine from the body. This catheter is left in place until the patient is able to respond to things going on around him. The catheter is then removed, and the individual is encouraged to try to empty his own bladder.

During the next 2 to 3 days the patient begins passing urine (voiding) on his own, and a "voiding schedule" is established. The time span between voidings is noted and used to plan the bladder retraining program. This program helps reestablish a normal pattern of urinary elimination. Any bladder problems that may be present, such as incontinence or retention, can also be observed at this time.

Whether the patient is bedridden or able to get up to go to the bathroom, certain measures should be taken when bladder problems exist. Allowing as much privacy as possible for toileting helps in relaxation. It is important to make sure an individual's balance is good enough for him to be left alone: Good balance decreases the chance of injury due to falls.

Dressing the patient in his own clothes helps him maintain his feeling of personal dignity as well as his individuality. Men may use Velcro instead of a zipper in their pants, and women should avoid wearing panties.

It is important that the patient drink at least one glass of fluid an hour between the hours of 8 a.m. and 8 p.m. (total fluid intake of 2.5 to 3.0 quarts in a 24-hour period). Fluid is restricted between 8 p.m. and 8 a.m., so as to decrease the chance of night urination (nocturia). Fluids that increase the need to void, such as caffeine-containing beverages and alcohol, should be avoided.

Incontinence

Incontinence is the main symptom of an "uninhibited neurogenic bladder." Other names used to describe the same condition are hypertonic, automatic, reflex, or spastic bladder.

In persons with an uninhibited bladder the messages from the brain to the bladder that regulate the inhibition of contractions of bladder muscles are blocked. When this blockage occurs, the bladder's capacity is reduced. A small degree of stretching, then, can cause the muscles that control the passage of urine from the bladder to the outside of the body to automatically open, and the bladder empties without any conscious effort by the individual. The bladder muscles, because of a lack of messages from the brain, are overactive and contract with extreme force.

Usually the individual with an uninhibited bladder can feel when his bladder contracts, but the feeling comes almost at the same time as its emptying. Thus he is aware of the need to empty his bladder but is unable to "hold it" until he can get to the bathroom. Most of these patients experience the need to (a) empty the bladder immediately (urgency), (b) void or empty the bladder often (frequency), and (c) empty the bladder during the night (nocturia). If the stroke patient has an uninhibited neurogenic bladder, management is aimed at stimulating and emptying the bladder before overstretching the bladder muscles.

Specific guidelines for managing incontinence in the stroke patient who is bedridden are outlined below.

1. Use the "voiding schedule" established after the catheter is removed, predicting when voiding may occur, and offer the bedpan or urinal before it happens. If the patient was noted to be voiding every 3 to 4 hours, establish a "timed voiding" schedule by offering the bedpan or urinal every 2 to 3 hours. This timing prevents overstretching of the bladder muscle, which causes incontinence.

2. Always be alert to signals that indicate the need to empty

the bladder and respond quickly to get the bedpan or urinal. Some of the signals used to indicate the need to urinate if unable to verbalize are as follows.

Gestures, such as motioning to the perineum
Facial expressions, such as a grimace
Pulling at clothes
Sudden agitation
Attempt to get out of bed
Sweating about the face

If the stroke patient is able to understand, try to work out *one* signal that can be easily remembered by him and let all those caring for him know what the signal is and what it means.

3. Encourage the patient to sit as upright as possible while attempting to void, as it increases intraabdominal pressure and aids in the flow of urine from the bladder. Have him push forward over the suprapubic, or bladder, area (Credé's maneuver) while he attempts to void.

4. Before the patient goes to bed for the night, the following are suggested guidelines to follow.

Offer the bedpan or urinal and have him attempt to void.
Do make sure that a call bell of some sort is where the patient can get it, and be sure he knows how to call if help is needed.
The bedpan or urinal should be close at hand if needed.
Above all, be alert to the patient's needs during the night and respond quickly if needed (if necessary, set clock for around 3 a.m. and offer him the opportunity to void).

On the other hand, if the patient is able to get up to go to the bathroom, these guidelines should be noted.

1. Use an elevated toilet seat to relieve stress or fatigue caused by a low toilet seat.

2. Have the patient use stimulation techniques to help "trigger" voiding.

Use Credé's maneuver (see above).

Pinch or stroke the inner thigh.

Massage or gently rub the abdomen in a clockwise motion.

Gently pull the pubic hairs.

Pour warm water over the perineum.

3. At bedtime, place a walker or cane at the patient's bedside. Also, turn the night light on and assist the patient as needed.

The bladder "retraining" program is always individualized to fit the life style of the patient. All responses (voidings) and incontinence are noted and modifications in the "retraining" program made as necessary.

Medications may be prescribed by the physician to help in this "retraining" program. Most of the time anticholinergic drugs are used because they relax the bladder muscles, enabling the bladder to hold more urine. This type of medicine, along with the "timed voidings," decreases the chance of overstretching the bladder, which is responsible for the incontinence. Examples of anticholinergic drugs are oxybutynin (Ditropan) and hyoscyamine (Cysto-Spaz).

Most of the time "retraining" eliminates urinary "accidents," and the individual has no need to worry about "embarrassments" happening. However, some patients still like to use something to make them more secure in case of an "accident." Men usually wear a condom attached to their penis by means of adhesive strips. The condom is attached rather loosely so as not to cut off the blood supply to the penis, and it is removed at least once a day so the penis can be washed thoroughly to prevent irritation. During the day a big bag connected to the condom is worn, but at night the condom is attached to a bedside drainage bag. Women wear rubber panties and extra padding to prevent "accidents." Diapers are worn by both men and women. Most of these articles are available at pharmacies or drugstores. If incontinence persists, the physician should be notified. Sometimes a permanent catheter can be inserted during the time a further urinary workup is being done.

Urinary incontinence may lead to another problem: skin breakdown. It is important to keep the skin healthy, which can be done by eating a well-balanced diet, maintaining an adequate fluid intake, keeping the skin intact and lubricated with natural oils, and making sure the skin has an adequate blood supply.

Good personal hygiene with special attention to the perineum and rectal areas is important. Use mild soap and bathe the entire body every day, as well as the perineal and rectal areas after each time there is incontinence. Dry the skin gently and thoroughly. Lotions and creams may be applied to help keep the skin healthy and in good tone. Remember: "An ounce of prevention is worth a pound of cure." Good hygiene is important in order to prevent the ammonia in urine from irritating and breaking down the skin. If a breakdown occurs, notify the physician at once.

Retention

Retention is the main symptom of a motor paralytic bladder. Other names used to describe the same condition are hypotonic, flaccid, autonomous, atonic, and nonreflexic bladder.

In the person with a motor paralytic bladder there is a blockage of the messages from the brain to the bladder that regulate the involuntary contractions of the bladder muscles. Urine then builds up in the bladder, stretching its muscles to or beyond their limit. This overstretching continues until there is enough pressure in the bladder to force small amounts of urine from the bladder (overflow incontinence). The muscles in the bladder, because of the lack of messages from the brain, are limp and cannot contract with enough force to push all the urine out of the bladder.

Usually the individual with a paralytic bladder cannot feel when his bladder is full and does not void, or if he does he passes only a dribble. If there continues to be a buildup of urine, increased pressure forces the urine back up into the kidneys (reflux). Thus if the patient constantly passes small amounts of urine or dribbles urine, management is aimed at keeping the bladder empty of urine, preventing dribbling or reflux.

Management for the individual still bedridden is as follows.

1. Offer a bedpan or urinal.
2. If he is unable to void, try stimulation techniques.
3. If the individual voids, measure the amount of urine passed and then catheterize him to remove any remaining (residual) urine from the bladder.
4. If the amount of urine obtained upon catheterization is more than one-half glass, an intermittent catheterization regimen should be started.
5. If the individual is unable to void, catheterize him and begin the intermittent program (usually catheterizing every 4 hours around the clock).
6. The patient and his family should be instructed in the catheterization technique.
7. Allow privacy for catheterization and do it in a manner that does not embarrass the individual.
8. Let the patient know that after the intermittent catheterization program has gone on for a while the bladder may be "triggered" and so begin to empty on a regular schedule.

Medications may be prescribed by a physician to help in the "retraining" program. Urecholine is often used as it increases the contraction ability of the bladder muscles that aid in its emptying.

The individual affected by a stroke and experiencing dribbling may wish to wear protective devices between catheterizations in order to prevent the possibility of embarrassing "accidents." The same devices used for incontinence may be used here. Skin breakdown may also be a problem with a paralytic bladder, so good skin care is necessary, as it is with the uninhibited bladder.

Overall, most bladder problems are temporary and clear as

the brain compensates for the damage done by the stroke. Normal bladder control usually returns to the individual affected by a stroke. Even if the problem does not totally clear, management of these urinary problems enables the individual to live a normal life with few limitations.

Complications

Anytime there is a variation from normal bladder functioning, complications are possible. These complications are easily recognized, and there are methods to both prevent and manage them.

Infection

The definition of infection in this context is the presence of bacteria in the urine. Bladder infections may result from overstretching of the bladder, large amounts of urine left in the bladder, or improper personal hygiene.

Signs and symptoms of such infections include: cloudy, foul-smelling urine; mucus in the urine; blood in the urine; a sudden increase in the amount of urine left in the bladder; burning of the urinary opening (meatus) while passing urine; the need to empty the bladder frequently; and fever.

Prevention of bladder infections requires certain measures.

1. Make sure there is adequate fluid intake (2.5 to 3.0 quarts of fluid per day).

2. Maintain an adequate daily output of urine (2.5 quarts per day).

3. Keep the urine acidic (drink Kool-aid and cranberry juice; take vitamin C, 500 mg four times a day).

4. Avoid fluids that make urine alkaline (milk, citrus juice, carbonated drinks).

5. Avoid overstretching the bladder (empty the bladder often; never allow it to fill with more than 300 to 400 cc or 2.0 to 2.5 cups of urine).

6. Use good hygiene (wash the perineal area thoroughly, especially around the urinary opening).

Urinary Stones

Urinary stones represent calcium buildup in the kidneys and bladder. They are caused by alkaline urine, inadequate fluid intake, or both.

Signs and symptoms of urinary stones include: bloody urine; eggshell-like flakes or particles in the urine; and pain in the suprapubic, or bladder, area or in the low back area above the hips.

Steps that can be taken to prevent their formation include: ensuring an adequate fluid intake (2.5 to 3.0 quarts per day); keeping the urine acidic; keeping the patient active; and limiting the intake of foods high in calcium (dairy products).

If any of these signs and symptoms are noted in the individual with a bladder problem, notify a physician. He can work with the family to treat the complications and reinforce the ways by which they can be prevented.

BOWEL PROBLEMS

Bowel problems seen after a stroke are usually the result of immobility, decreased fluid intake, and a nutritionally inadequate diet. The problem is either constipation or diarrhea.

A thorough history of prestroke bowel habits is obtained. This history should provide the answers needed to formulate a bowel "retraining" program. The information needed includes:

1. Frequency of bowel movements
2. Usual time of bowel movements
3. Prior reliance on laxatives or enemas
4. History of diarrhea or constipation

By using the information obtained from the prestroke bowel

history, an individualized "retraining" program can be started. The post-stroke life style is taken into consideration when planning the "retraining" program.

A set time is established for the passage (elimination) of the bowels. Based on the life style the individual affected by stroke expects to have when he arrives back home, the designated time for the bowel movement is either in the morning after breakfast or in the evening after dinner. These times are chosen to take advantage of the normal bowel reflexes that help in the elimination of solid body waste (feces).

The bowel "retraining" program should be started with a clean bowel, which is accomplished by emptying the bowel with an enema. Privacy is provided, and all procedures are done in such a way as to promote comfort. Relaxation is encouraged in order to prevent excessive tightening of the bowel muscles.

The day after the cleansing enema, at the established time set for the bowel movement, a suppository is given. The suppository should be at room temperature and is inserted past the rectal sphincter or muscle. Always position the suppository against the bowel lining, not in the feces. Inserting the suppository into fecal material defeats its purpose, making it of no value.

If the patient is able to get out of bed, let him go to the bathroom to move his bowels. If he is still bedridden, elevate him to as near sitting as possible. This positioning is important as sitting increases intraabdominal pressure and aids in elimination. Leaning forward, massaging the abdomen in a clockwise motion, lifting buttocks off the toilet seat with hands, stroking thighs, and drinking a cup of hot fluid help stimulate bowel elimination.

After an adequate bowel movement, the perineal area is cleansed thoroughly using warm, soapy water, rinsed, and dried. Good hygiene helps prevent skin irritation, which can lead to skin ulcers or breakdown.

A suppository is then given every other day at the designated time. This regimen gets the bowel into the "habit" of emptying at a set time. After several weeks of the "retraining" program, the bowel may be so "retrained" that it automatically empties itself without the aid of a suppository. Often by just using stimulation techniques the individual can experience a good bowel movement. It is best to achieve retraining with as little mechanical or medical means as possible.

In order to have a good bowel "retraining" program, constipation and diarrhea must be prevented and regularity promoted. This pattern is important so the individual can lead a life that is "accident" free and not be constantly worried about being embarrassed. Ways to prevent constipation and diarrhea are discussed in the next sections.

Constipation

Constipation is the infrequent or difficult elimination of feces. It is usually due to lifelong habits but can also be due to breakdown in the nervous and hormonal systems. This breakdown may lead to a loss of feeling (sensation) and control of the bowel, rectum, and muscles of that area, and the stroke patient therefore may not have the sensation of bowel fullness. Thus there is a period of days between bowel movements, and the feces, when passed, are hard and dry.

The management of constipation is as follows.

1. Inform the patient and his family of some of the signs that indicate a bowel movement is needed. These signs include the following.

Abdominal enlargement (distention)
Rumbling sounds from abdomen
Passage of gas (flatus)
Nausea
Spasms in lower abdomen

2. Add bulk or roughage to the diet. This bulk increases pressure needed in the bowel to help pass feces through the digestive tract. The best way to add bulk is through a well-balanced diet. Some of the foods that are needed are the following.

Raw vegetables (lettuce, carrots)

Long-fiber vegetables (celery, cabbage, greens, kale)

Red meats (pork, beef, liver): high in thiamine (vitamin B_1) which improves elimination

Fish

Poultry

Whole fruits with skins intact (apples, peaches, grapes)

Stewed or dried fruits (apricots, dates, figs, prunes) (Prunes draw water from the body into the feces and act as an irritant to the bowel lining.)

Beans

Enriched grains, dark breads, whole wheat bread, whole grain cereals rich in thiamine (vitamin B_1). (These foods are high in cellulose, which is not totally digested by the body and therefore adds bulk to the bowel.)

Foods to be avoided are as follows.

Foods high in fat

Milk products (contain casein, which constipates)

Chocolate

Tea (contains tannic acid, which constipates)

3. It is important to not self-medicate for constipation (over-the-counter laxatives, enemas, or home remedies). The laxatives lead to bowel dependency, and enemas cause over-stretching of the bowel, producing loss of muscle control. Self-medication decreases the effectiveness of the "retraining" program.

4. It is essential that the patient have an adequate intake of fluids (2.5 to 3.0 quarts per day). Moisture aids in softening feces and keeps the bowel lining moist in order to help the passage of feces.

5. Increasing activity and mobility help build better muscle strength in the abdomen. Strength is important, as good muscles help push feces out of the body.

6. Prune juice (4 ounces) can be given either the evening before a scheduled morning bowel movement or the morning before a scheduled evening bowel movement.

7. Relaxation is encouraged to prevent muscle contraction in the abdomen and bowel that might stop elimination.

Relative to item 5, above, there may also be problems with muscle tone or with the rectal and anal openings. Such problems may cause the body to be unable to pass feces from it even if constipation is not the problem. Medical or mechanical help may be needed to correct this situation. These measures should be used only on the order of a physician, who can determine the proper method to use.

Medical Intervention

Bulk formers may be given. These substances add material to the intestines, giving them a fullness, which triggers elimination of feces. Natural bulk formers are bran, fruits, and vegetables with seeds. Commercially, Metamucil is available. A lot of fluid should be taken with these substances, as there is a tendency for them to draw water from the feces.

Peristaltic stimulators may also be useful. They increase the wave-like motions of the bowel, which pushes feces from body. Examples of these agents are danthron (Doxidan), docusate sodium (Peri-Colace), and docusate potassium (Dialose Plus).

Stool softeners and *detergent stool softeners*, which cause retention of water and breakdown of fat in the bowel, keep feces soft and passable. Docusate calcium (Surfak), docusate sodium (Colace), and docusate potassium (Dialose) are examples.

Magnesia stops absorption of water, causing increased bulk in the bowel.

Suppositories or *chemical irritants* are sometimes prescribed. Glycerin, for example, stimulates nerve endings in the intestinal wall and thereby causes elimination. Bisacodyl (Dulcolax) irritates the lining of bowel, causing fluid buildup in the bowel, which acts as a lubricant for elimination. Carbon dioxide, or Vacuett, forms a gas that creates pressure in the bowel, aiding elimination.

Mechanical Intervention

Enemas irritate the bowel lining and add bulk, thereby aiding elimination. Examples are the various Fleet enemas, soap suds enemas, oil retention enemas, and plain tap water enemas.

Digital stimulation is performed by gently inserting a finger into the rectum and then moving it in a circular or back-and-forth motion, thereby stimulating elimination of feces.

Digital removal may also be tried. A finger is gently inserted into rectum, and feces are manually removed from the bowel. This method is often used to remove hardened feces that are blocking the passage of softer feces (a condition known as impaction).

Diarrhea

Diarrhea is the repeated passage of small amounts of loose or watery feces from the bowel. Some patients may experience this problem after stroke, and it may be due to several factors. Some of the causes of diarrhea and their management are given in Table 3.

The overall objective of both bladder and bowel management programs is the maintenance of dignity and self-esteem of the individual affected by stroke. Patience and hard work

TABLE 3. *Causes of diarrhea and their management*

Cause	Management
Intake of indiscriminate food source (pizza, spicy Mexican food)	Avoid the foods.
Intake of indiscriminate fluid (alcohol)	Avoid alcohol.
Overmedication with stool softeners or oral laxatives	Stop stool softener or oral laxative temporarily; readjust dosage and frequency to maintain firm but soft feces.
Antibiotic therapy	May use Mycostatin in conjunction with antibiotics. Medications to slow elimination may be given in order to decrease diarrhea [diphenoxylate (Lomotil), kaolin (Kaopectate), Lactinex]. Foods known to constipate may be encouraged for a while (cheese, milk, chocolate).
Impaction	Try to remove by digital manipulation. If unsuccessful, give a suppository to move the impaction down to where it can be reached, if not eliminated. If impaction is still present, give an oral laxative and enema as ordered by the physician.

on the part of the individual and his family determine the effectiveness of these "retraining" programs. The individual's being able to live a normal life without fear of embarrassing "accidents" is the greatest reward.

14

Sexual Problems

Nancy Crater

Everyone, regardless of age, sex, or physical limitations, is a sexual being and needs sexual expression and intimate relationships. "Sexuality" is not only the sex drive but a combination of biological genes (anatomy), psychological feelings (how we feel about ourselves), and social input (how society expects us to be). Sexuality therefore varies among people depending on the influence of these three factors.

After a stroke the individual and his family try to establish a life style that is as normal as possible in regard to the life they had before. One of their main concerns is whether sex will continue to be a part of their life. Be reassured: *Sex does exist after a stroke*. This fact is important to remember, as most people tend to ignore or deny the sexual needs of the individual affected by stroke.

Usually there is no physical reason for changes in sexual interest or desire after a stroke. The sudden interruption of normal sexual activity may cause some confusion. These interruptions occur because after a stroke the individual is more attentive to his physical reactions during the performance of sex. The various aspects involved in the normal sex act and how stroke and aging change these responses in men and women are described as follows.

177

DESIRE OR LIBIDO

During early adolescence the sexual desire of boys is strong. It is greatly influenced by hormonal, psychological, and sociological factors. The production of testosterone, peer pressure, and the view society has about virile young men greatly increases a young man's desire for sexual activity.

As a man ages, there is a decrease in the production of testosterone, a decrease in the need to prove virility to others, and a more negative view from society (for instance, the references to "dirty old men").

In contrast, during early adolescence the desire of girls is less strong than that of boys. It also is greatly influenced by hormonal, psychological, and sociological factors. The production of testosterone is outweighed by the production of estrogen and progesterone, which cause a decrease in the stimulating effects of testosterone. Peer pressure is still a strong influence, as for boys. Most of the time, society's view about the sexual activities expected by women, however, overcomes peer pressure. As a woman ages, the estrogen and progesterone decrease and the stimulating effects of testosterone become prominent, increasing desire, or libido. The emotional aspects of menopause (decreased sexual worth and gender identity) battle the increase of desire. This ongoing battle may result in either increased or decreased desire, depending on hormone levels.

ERECTION

The older a man gets the more noticeable are the physical changes in regard to erection. These changes can be caused by decreased testosterone levels or emotional stresses. The man often finds that more physical manipulation and longer foreplay is needed to achieve an erection. He finds that mental thoughts or pictures do not help him obtain his erection as they once did. These changes can greatly decrease his desire to attempt an erection. When erection is achieved, the man often experiences a decrease in orgasmic urgency and sexual haste.

Increased vaginal lubrication is equivalent to an erection in women. As women age, they notice that the glands responsible for lubrication take longer to be effective. Furthermore, there is much less lubrication than before. The tissue around and inside the vaginal opening thins and becomes more fragile because of the reduced estrogen production. These changes often lead to painful intercourse, causing the woman to fear or avoid sexual activity.

EJACULATION

As men age there is a decrease in the feeling of imminent ejaculation, in the sensation of ejaculation, and in the amount and thickness of seminal fluid. These changes are usually caused by enlargement of the prostate gland. Aging also causes an increase in the time span between sexual functioning.

Women may find that the fragility and shrinking of vaginal tissue cause pain during intercourse. Thoughts of the pain associated with sex usually outweigh the desire for orgasm.

It is important that men and women understand the bodily changes due to aging. Using this knowledge, they can decide if the sexual changes are a result of normal aging or are caused by the stroke. Sexual problems are often due to physical and emotional causes.

Depression

Depression is the frequent cause of many sexual problems (decreased desire, shorter foreplay, less caring gestures, fatigue, and erectile dysfunction). The depression is often a side effect of pressures bearing on the individual's mind. Some of the problems that are worrisome can include the patient's difficulty in moving or feeling a part of the body due to motor or sensory loss. In addition, difficulty in understanding or communicating one's thoughts and needs can be frustrating. Also, physical problems such as bowel and bladder incontinence may limit sexual activity.

The stroke patient may feel he is not an attractive person anymore. This assessment leads to a feeling that he is not worth loving. Lowered self-esteem can lead to a decrease in desire. Thus it is essential that the stroke patient be reassured and shown that he is loved and desired. He must be made to realize that touching, holding, sharing closeness, and living with him are still important. It is important to stress that regardless of whether he is in the mood for sex, he is loved. If he cannot perform the sexual act, let him know that just sharing the intimacy of being alone with him is satisfying. If something is not done to help this lowered esteem, impotence or frigidity may occur.

Both the patient and the mate must learn to be open and honest with each other. They must share their feelings, fears, and triumphs. There must be an open channel of communication about everything between them.

Fear

Fear produces great stress on the stroke patient and the mate. Fear that sex will cause another stroke is paramount in their minds. Such fear can cause a decrease in the desire for sexual intimacy. The activity involved in sex is unlikely to cause another stroke. A person's blood pressure does not increase much more during sex than it does during normal exertions of daily living. Most physicians believe that individuals affected by a stroke may resume sexual activities as soon as they want to. Usually there are no limits placed on the intensity with which they can resume their sexual role. Sexual expression is good for all. It is good to be active in sex—as it is to be active in other activities of daily living. Fear that the patient is no longer a sexual being and fear of inability to perform can cause difficulty with performance.

Medications

Medications such as antidepressants, antihypertensives, antiadrenergics, and anticholinergics may cause side effects that affect sexual function (impotence, decreased penile erections, ejaculatory problems, and decreased sexual interest). If problems are noted and do not go away, contact the doctor. He can check the patient and may be able to change or adjust the medicines. If a medical cause cannot be found, however, it is important to help the patient realize that sex is not an all-or-nothing experience. As much loving and sharing can occur without intercourse as can with the actual vaginal-penile penetration. It is important for the stroke patient to learn to let others love him.

Role Change

Role change after a stroke can also lead to sexual problems. Often the patient feels useless as he is no longer able to perform the duties he once did. He may feel that he is a burden on his mate. The great dependency on his mate and the loss of control over his life may lead to a decrease in sexual activity. Reassurance should be given that he is still a functioning part of the family. Explain that the stability he gives to the family is worth more than any other duty he could do. After a stroke the patient may have many adjustments to make (sexual identity, sexual role, body image, and self-esteem). The mate should be aware of these adjustments and give him as much support as possible.

The partner also may experience difficulty with role change. Being asked to help meet many of the patient's needs sometimes makes it difficult to switch from caregiver to lover. This problem may need to be discussed not only with the partner but with a therapist as well. Learning to express one's self in different roles can, however, prove challenging. It is helpful to be eager to explore ways to lessen frustration surrounding this issue. Difficulties are compounded when both partners experience adjustment problems.

Physical Limitations

Physical limitations after a stroke may pose some problems so far as sex is concerned. Both patient and partner may have to learn to be uninhibited in thought and actions. Experimentation of new sexual positions may be necessary. Lying on one's side or reversing positions may be needed in order to decrease the effort required to participate in active sexual activity. There are several books available on alternate positionings for sexual intercourse. The couple must be aggressive about obtaining information on how to exercise their sexuality.

Changes from the previous normal sexual expression are a valid concern for both partners and should be discussed with all involved. In order to have a reasonable discussion a counselor needs to know the individuals' values. Reassurance is given that all concerns and questions are normal.

Exploring new areas of pleasure is encouraged. It is important that sex never become routine, so it is well to try new things. Sexuality is the responsibility of both individuals, and what they do with it is up to them. A balance of giving and receiving between the two individuals is necessary for a good sexual relationship. Sexual expression should be regarded as an individual experience without rules or score cards. There are many ways to give and receive sexual pleasure. Satisfaction is possible for anyone who wishes to seek it.

If problems still exist after each partner has given 100%, counseling by a certified sexual therapist may be needed. Further evaluation by a physician may also be required to rule out a physical problem.

Contraception is an issue that needs to be discussed with the couple if the woman is within child-bearing years. Precautions should be taken unless pregnancy is desired. A gynecologist should be consulted in order to discuss methods of birth control.

Sexuality in the individual affected by stroke is extremely important. Understanding underlying stresses and physical problems that cause temporary sexual inadequacies helps the couple maintain their dignity as sexual beings—and dignity is one of the most important aspects of the sexual gambit.

15

Finding Help Along the Way

Once the patient's condition is stable, both he and his family become aware that their lives have changed as a result of the stroke. Some individuals can deal with these changes more easily than others. Yet for most there is a feeling of frustration and disappointment if all the patient's needs are not met by the family members. Trying to meet all the demands can be difficult, and assistance with handling some of them becomes essential for the well-being of all. "Who can help?" and "Where do we go to find this help?" are questions commonly asked.

Those who can best assist the patient and family initially are the health care personnel who have been with them throughout the hospitalization. By having had day-by-day contact, these individuals can best determine what services may be needed. For instance, the physician and nurses can determine if there is need for a home health nurse, and the physical therapist may suggest continued therapy sessions on an outpatient basis. Does the patient require speech therapy? Are renovations needed in the home? What financial services are available to assist with these needs? The hospital staff can direct the patient and family to specialists in these areas. Communities differ in the resources available to the patient and family. The most common services are discussed here.

SPECIAL SERVICES

Most communities provide special services, such as home visitation programs offered by the local health department.

Public health nurses follow patients for a specified time, supplying them with physical and emotional needs.

Adult day care centers are available in some communities. They enable individuals who require minimal care to stay in a facility for specified hours of the day. Generally, family members may need to work or want someone to observe the individual for a few hours while they attend to other matters. Cost is usually a set fee, and meals are provided if desired. Social and recreational services are provided at most centers.

Meals on Wheels is another community function that delivers hot meals for senior citizens or home-bound individuals who are unable to provide adequate nourishment for themselves.

Transportation needs are met in some areas by making buses and vans available. This service provides more freedom for the patient and his family. Shopping, seeing the doctor, or visiting a recreational center, even if one needs a wheelchair, can be a viable option with the use of a transit system.

Changes in the structure of the home environment may be discussed with an architect or an agency such as the one referred to in Chapter 10. Such changes may make living at home comfortable for both the patient and his family.

The local mental health center or area churches are sources of counseling for the patient or family. Psychologists, psychiatrists, or both can also be found in local communities. The patient's physician may be able to direct the patient and his family to one with expertise in the area needed. The area of mental health problems is often overlooked because it is often easier for others to concern themselves with physical needs than emotional ones. However, with available resources this problem should not occur.

Some areas offer a daily telephone reassurance program in which individuals can call for a message of encouragement. Local "hot lines" are also available that provide information on all the services in a particular area.

Recreational facilities are becoming more popular and are

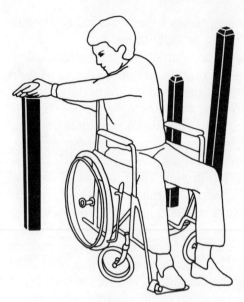

FIG. 50. Twisting reach.

a valuable resource. Swimming, arts and crafts, and sports conducted while in a wheelchair are popular activities for the stroke survivor. All are therapeutic on a physical and emotional basis. Many programs and instructors are available to assist in these activities and more.

One interesting activity is the wheelchair sports course. It is being promoted by the National Fitness Campaign located at 50 Fran Street, Suite 265, San Francisco, California 94133. This company has made it possible for individuals requiring the use of a wheelchair to engage in exercises not only for strengthening and stretching muscle groups but for fun as well. Family members often find the course useful as well, as they walk beside the patient and get additional exercise themselves.

Courses are made up of stations with specific exercises to be done at each one. Figures 50, 51, and 52 show exercises that have been modified for the stroke patient. A useful aim is to exercise the affected side as well as the nonaffected one.

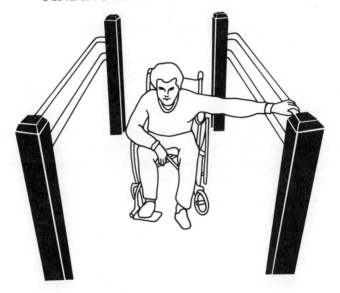

FIG. 51. Side wide grip run.

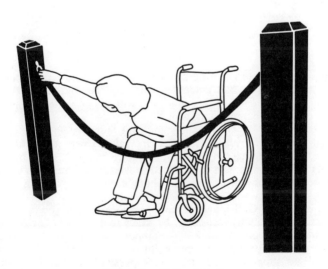

FIG. 52. Side stretch.

More information on the sports course may be obtained by writing to the address above.

Vocational rehabilitation can assist individuals who want to return to work or to pursue an education. It is difficult for some stroke patients to continue doing the work they did because they have lost their previous abilities. Trained counselors at vocational rehabilitation offices can be of assistance in finding work the patient can do. Sometimes less physical exertion and fewer hours are the only changes necessary. For instance, a former mail carrier may now need a desk job. Furthermore, he may even find this job as great a challenge and equally rewarding.

A few patients who return to work encounter difficulty in doing so. It appears that once the patient returns to work on a permanent basis, he stands the chance of losing some of his Medicare benefits. These benefits are a must for most patients, helping them with medical bills and giving support for any problems they encounter down the road. Most companies do not insure these individuals because of their present health conditions. This type of disincentive therefore makes many not want to return to employment. They have no choice but to live on Medicare and/or disability. Such was the case with M.G.

M.G. was 25 years old when he had a stroke caused by a faulty valve in his heart. Although he had graduated from college with a degree in art design, he found little use for his education with his disabilities. The weakness in his arms hindered his drawing abilities.

Five years later M.G. had made significant recovery and was eager to get out into the world again. He wanted especially to meet people and make new friends. He volunteered for work at a local hospital, handling his assignments well. He was then approached to work in an area with duties he was quite capable of performing. The thought of making a salary and accepting responsibility was exciting to him.

Unfortunately, M.G. discovered that upon accepting his job he would be ineligible for his disability insurance. He knew that he could not depend on this job alone for his entire future. It was impossible to predict that he would not need Medicare benefits at some point. In later years his family might not be able to support him as they were presently doing. Therefore he decided to continue his volunteer work and turned down the opportunity.

There are many other individuals who have encountered this type of problem. A leading advocate for the handicapped and who is trying to reverse this situation is Deborah Crouch McKeithan, founder and president of HOW (Handicapped Organized Women).

Ms. McKeithan has multiple sclerosis and epilepsy, has had a stroke, and is legally blind. All of these problems, and she is just in her early thirties. Yet Ms. McKeithan has been determined to overcome these disabilities. She founded HOW with the purpose of returning to work and eager to help others. HOW is composed of physically disabled women who are 18 years of age or older. Each year the members are required to perform two volunteer projects that help the community in some way. By sharing experiences, each member of HOW can find a good support system with the group.

Unfortunately, if she accepted salary for her job as the president of this organization, Ms. McKeithan would be ineligible for Social Security Disability Insurance. Being unable to receive a social security check was not a problem but being unable to have Medicare insurance would be. If her health were to get worse in the future, she would be unable to qualify for Medicare again. This issue is an important one. Ms. McKeithan is therefore spending much of her time trying to convince Congress to pass legislation that allows individuals with disabilities to work and purchase Medicare insurance on a sliding scale according to their income. Information about financial sources such as those we have discussed can be obtained through local departments of social services. Many people are eligible for services but do not utilize them because they are not aware of their existence.

FINANCIAL SOURCES

In the United States persons 65 years of age and older are eligible for Medicare; some who are under 65 and disabled may also qualify. Medicare is a health insurance program operated by the Social Security Administration (SSA). It assists with payments for hospitalization, therapy, and medical equipment. Social Security offices can give information about services covered by Medicare and the extent to which they will pay.

Medicaid is a program funded by federal, state, and local taxes. It operates on the state level and assists individuals who are unable to pay for medical needs. In order to qualify for this program, one must apply and be interviewed at the Department of Social Services. Usually personal health insurance and Medicare benefits are used before Medicaid can be put into effect. However, exceptions are sometimes made that enable both sources to be used.

Along with Medicare, patients 65 and older may be eligible for supplemental security income (SSI). Other individuals, such as the blind or disabled under 65, may qualify if they require financial assistance. The extent of disability must be confirmed by medical personnel.

Social Security disability payments (as previously discussed) are available to those who meet eligibility requirements. To qualify an individual must have worked at least 5 of the last 10 years and is unable to return to work for at least a year after a stroke owing to disabilities that exist as a result of that stroke. Applications can be obtained at the local SSA office. The SSA in turn determines if the patient's medical condition makes him eligible.

Other sources, such as retirement checks from the SSA, are available to individuals at the age of 62. The amount an individual receives is determined by how long he worked at jobs that required him to pay into the social security system.

STROKE CLUBS/SUPPORT AGENCIES

Another support group for all stroke patients and their families is the Stroke Club, sponsored by the Easter Seal Society. Stroke clubs have the purpose of bringing together individuals who have had a stroke along with their family members so they can share concerns, find ways to solve problems they may be experiencing, and offer support to each other.

In addition to developing a close network of friendships among its members, the Stroke Club may also serve as an avenue for providing information on stroke and/or resources that offer help with various problems. For instance, a member of the home visitation program may be invited to speak on the nursing care available to patients. At another meeting, a member of the city transportation department may want to inform members of services they provide. Newsletters are usually sent on a monthly basis informing members of latest events and upcoming projects. Most clubs meet once monthly.

Many members of the Stroke Club in one area spoke of their initial feelings of uneasiness with being together with strangers in a group. Some thought that their difficulty with speaking or ambulating was easier to handle around family than others. Yet it was astonishing to them that being with others experiencing similar feelings made the situation less noticeable. One man spoke of his excitement on coming to the meetings because most of his former friends did not visit him or invite him to their homes anymore. Now he feels accepted by others and has made contact with people he might never have attempted to get to know. Belonging to a Stroke Club can be rewarding to the patient and his family. All it takes are a few interested individuals who are willing to take the necessary steps to get a club started. Most states have an Easter Seal Society that has a toll-free number to call to ask for assistance on how to begin. One can also write for this information as well as information about books and pamphlets on stroke at the following address.

National Easter Seal Society
2023 W. Ogden Avenue
Chicago, Illinois 60612

There is a charge of 50 cents for the reference list.

The American Heart Association at the national, state, and local levels is instrumental in providing educational materials on stroke to the general public. Local agencies in some areas also sponsor blood pressure monitoring programs that screen for high blood pressure, a risk factor of stroke and heart disease.

The National Stroke Association, located in Denver, Colorado, is an organization founded specifically to assist survivors of stroke and to educate their families and the general public about stroke. Newsletters and information packets on various aspects of stroke are sent to those interested.

It is hoped that the resources mentioned in this chapter are useful in helping to meet the particular needs of the patient and his family. Most of these suggestions can make caring for the patient at home more manageable.

However, there are situations in which placement in a health care facility is a more feasible solution. This arrangement can be a temporary or a permanent situation. For instance, the family may need to place the patient in a facility until the home environment is made ready for the patient. Situations may also occur in which the patient's condition improves over time and the family desires to bring him home.

If placement is permanent, it may take time for the patient and his family to adjust to the change. Both need to be able to express their feelings about the situation. There may be guilt on the part of the family as well as anger from the patient regarding placement. Talking with a therapist or a counselor may enable both to understand and accept the decision better. Hopefully, by choosing a place with which both patient and family are comfortable some anxieties can be alleviated. The Social Service Department can make information on facilities available.

Knowledge of community resources makes any decision somewhat easier, whether it is where the family member will live, what financial help he will need, or what services he will require. Awareness of these sources of help makes the adjustment after stroke less difficult and changes in the future more acceptable.

16

Promising Research

There are dozens of exciting new research activities that hold promise for prevention of stroke and for better management of those unfortunates who suffer one. One area being explored is better ways to identify individuals at excess risk for stroke, so that proper steps can be taken to prevent it. Of course, anyone at any age may develop stroke, but some people are at far greater risk than others. The customary risk factors were described in Chapter 1, and it is to everyone's advantage to attempt to reduce these factors by adhering to proper habits for good health.

IDENTIFYING RISKS

There are means for detecting people who, despite their attempts at prevention, have increased risk for stroke. One way is to have individuals measure their own blood pressure. Home systems have been developed for self-measurement, but one difficulty is that these systems are erratic in behavior and require maintenance and adjustments. Furthermore, some individuals have arms that are either too fat or too thin for the cuff to measure pressure accurately. The technology will undoubtedly improve, and the measurement of blood pressure in small children will become routine.

Screening programs for detecting the early manifestations of arteriosclerosis in the arteries in the neck are being initiated using ultrasound technology. It is likely that the accuracy of this technology will continue to increase, and the technique will be widely available in the future, so that individuals can undergo these tests as readily as they undergo chest x-ray studies or electrocardiography.

TO TREAT OR NOT TO TREAT?

There is great controversy among the experts about what to do with individuals who are detected as having borderline blood pressure or arteriosclerosis in the arteries of the neck. After all, everyone grows old and eventually dies, so that some experts suggest, "Why not let nature take its course?" This pessimistic view is opposed by physicians who believe that disability and death should be postponed as long as possible, and that people deserve perfect health during their time on this earth. To be disabled by stroke often means to be dead on one side of the body, which is a disaster to be prevented by any means possible. Therefore techniques for keeping blood pressure under control, such as teaching relaxation, altering diet, taking a medication every day, are justifiable goals for researchers. Much effort is being made along these lines to identify methods that are useful for accomplishing the goal of normal blood pressure without requiring large investments of time and money or alteration of the individual's life style. Particularly useful would be a once-a-week or once-a-month medicine that keeps blood pressure normal without harmful side effects.

The question of what to do about atherosclerosis is more problematical because it requires larger changes in one's eating habits, which, even then, gives no guarantee of regression or of halting the progression of the disease. One current area of intense investigation is whether taking aspirin each day helps prevent heart attacks and strokes in those who have atherosclerosis. There is proof that aspirin reduces the risk of stroke and death in patients who are symptomatic with transient ischemic attacks, but there is no evidence at this moment that aspirin is useful for preventing strokes in those who have not yet developed symptoms. Although it seems reasonable to think that it would, the prospect of suggesting that individuals at risk be on a lifetime regimen of aspirin is not appropriate.

Research requires time and large numbers of individuals to participate in it, as well as an investment of large sums of money for the coordination of the activity and analysis of the data. Sometimes the studies produce surprising results by proving that something that everybody had thought effective was in actuality useless. Such is the case with the extracranial-to-intracranial bypass surgical procedure that held so much promise for providing new arterial blood supply to the brain after patients had had stroke. It required 8 years and an enormous financial investment to prove the ineffectual nature of this surgery, but it was well worth it because the annual cost of this operation in the United States had begun to exceed $10 million. Currently there is one ongoing clinical trial to determine if surgery for asymptomatic blockage of arteries in the neck can prevent further arterial blockage and if aspirin can prevent the progression of atherosclerosis.

REDUCING THE EFFECTS OF STROKE

Most important of all, research into new ways to reduce the effects of stroke once they have begun is moving along rapidly. Reducing the effects of stroke is one of the most important and yet one of the most difficult areas of research in which to work. It stands to reason that in order to reverse the progress of stroke, the individual must be kept in proper facilities. It is a shocking reality that many patients are not hospitalized quickly, and they are treated in a customary but not emergency manner by their physicians. As a consequence, one prospect for research is education—the need to change attitudes about emergency transportation of the individual with certain forms of stroke to the hospital by ground or air transportation.

Once having arrived at the medical center, immediate ascertainment of the location and type of problem is essential before therapy can be initiated. Emergency evaluation must be followed by several diagnostic tests (described in other chapters). If the problem is a hemorrhage into the brain, although there is much research, little can be done to reduce its effects or stop the flow during the acute phase. If the bleeding is a subarachnoid hemorrhage (that is, around the brain) the flow of blood may be stopped and the effects of the free blood within the subarachnoid space surrounding the brain can be reduced by still-experimental methods for making blood clot. Surgery is then directed against the bleeding site. Means for reducing the flow of blood include the use of substances that cause blood to clot and at times placing a balloon or tampon into the area of the bleeding and inflating it so that it plugs the hole.

In theory, there are two aspects of the emergency treatment of stroke. The first is to ensure that the blood vessels and the blood flowing through them perform their functions properly. In the case of hemorrhage the bleeding must be stopped, whereas in the case of a blood clot, such as embolism, the clot must be dissolved so that blood can flow through the artery again. The second aspect of the acute treatment of stroke is to protect the brain during the time the blood flow is not normal.

Research activities concerning the blood vessels and the blood itself fall into two categories: (a) what to do about blood that is escaping from the blood vessels (as with bleeding) and (b) what to do about arteries that are plugged by a blood clot leading to little blood flow into the brain.

Regarding the former problem, we have already discussed the possibility of plugging arterial bleeding sites by making the blood more coagulable, as well as using artificial tampons, or balloons, which can be placed at the site of the bleeding. With regard to the latter problem, certain chemicals, particularly a substance called tissue plasminogen activator, can be used to dissolve existing blood clots. The problem here is that when such a substance is given it may cause bleeding in other locations. Therefore, being investigated are techniques for threading a catheter through the artery to the spot where the clot is blocking the artery so that tiny quantities of plasminogen activator can be injected specifically at the site of the clot. The success of this method for local dissolution of clots has been encouraging.

For those arteries that are tightly stenosed (narrowed) by atherosclerosis, another avenue is being explored. Constricted arteries are being dilated with a balloon (deflated) that is floated in the bloodstream to the constriction and then inflated. As the balloon fills, it stretches the arterial wall and relieves the constriction. The danger here is that fragments of tissue are sometimes loosened from the arterial wall and are carried by the bloodstream to the brain, lodging there and causing a stroke. These two techniques are currently under experimental consideration and are exciting prospects for the future.

Protecting the brain during the acute attack has enormous theoretical potential, but the problem is that the very tissues that one needs to protect have lost the normal channels for blood flow, so that materials injected into the bloodstream may not get to where they are needed most. Certain measures are therefore taken to reduce the need of the tissue for oxygen and nutrients. Sedation of the patient and cooling of the tissue have been tried in this regard with variable degrees of success. Another method is to provide an excessive quantity of oxygen under pressure using a hyperbaric chamber or administering 100% oxygen. There are theoretical reasons why this method should work but practical reasons why it may not. Still another means is to use blood thinners, which keep blood from clotting and obstructing arteries that supply the brain. Another is to dilute the blood so that fewer red blood cells are flowing through the tissue; this technique makes the blood more liquid (reduces its viscosity) so that it flows more easily through the capillaries (tiny blood vessels), which remain open. All of these systems are currently under investigation with money supplied by the federal government and other research groups.

GEOGRAPHICAL DISTRIBUTION OF STROKE

Another area of promising research is concerned with the variable distribution of stroke on the basis of geography. One of the most intriguing enigmas of stroke research is the fact that stroke occurs less commonly at higher elevations than at the seacoasts of the world. This finding holds true not only for the United States but for other countries as well. Japan is an example. Whether it is true everywhere in the world is unknown, however. As stroke research becomes more sophisticated, there is more cognizance of this fact, and researchers are devoting time and energy to determining why this variation occurs. Answers to this question may provide clues that can be applied to populations at high risk.

There are those who believe that the reason stroke is more common in the lowlands is that people there might have a higher salt content in their diets or their drinking water. Others, however, believe that it relates to the exercise or, to a certain extent, to the change in barometric pressure. There is also interest in the fact that the frequency of stroke has a time distribution, occurring most commonly during the midmorning hours and less commonly during the afternoon, evening, and night. This finding does not seem to be specifically related to the fact that stroke may have occurred during sleep and is recognized only after one awakens, although this explanation is a possibility. Thus these intriguing findings lead us to believe that research in epidemiology and global pathology will be useful.

Bibliography

ARTICLES

1. DuFault, K. (1978): Urinary incontinence, U.S. and British nursing perceptive. *J. Gerontol. Nurs.*, 4(2):128–133.
2. Eisenberg, M. G. (1977): Psychological aspects of disability: a guide for the health care educator. *NLN Publ. League Exchange*, 114:1–32.
3. Johnson, J. (1980): Rehabilitative concepts of neurological bladder dysfunction. *Nurs. Clin. North Am.*, 15(2):223–230.
4. Psychological implications of a neurogenic bladder (1984): *Rehabil. Nurs.*, 9(4):35–37.
5. Robinson, R. G., Lipsey, J. R., and Price, T. R. (1985): Diagnosis and clinical management of post-stroke depression. *Psychosomatics*, 26:769–778.
6. Sexual changes in patients and partners following stroke (1985): *Rehabil. Nurs.*, 10(2):28–31.
7. Swartz, C. (1982): Hormones and depressive illness. *The Female Patient*, 7:32–33.

BOOKS

1. Anderson, F., Bardach, J., and Goodgold, J. (1979): *Sexuality and Neuromuscular Diseases*. Institute of Rehabilitation Medicine and the Muscular Dystrophy Association, New York.
2. Berkow, R. (1977): Neurogenic bladder. In: *Merck Man-

ual of Diagnosis and Treatment, 13th ed. Merck Sharp and Dohme Research Laboratories, Rahway, New Jersey.

3. Bray, G. P., and Clark, G. S., editors (1984): *A Stroke Family Guide and Resource*. Charles C Thomas, Springfield, Illinois.

4. Coker, L. H., and Toole, J. F. (1986): Assessment and rehabilitation of the patient recovering from stroke. In: *Mosby's Comprehensive Review of Critical Care 1986*, edited by D. Zschoche, 3rd ed., pp. 700–708. Mosby, St. Louis.

5. Crosby, W. H. (1982): The blood. In: *Better Homes and Gardens New Family Medical Guide*, edited by E. Keister Jr., pp. 89–117. Meredith Corporation, Des Moines.

6. Krusen, F. H., Kottke, F. J., and Ellwood, P. M., Jr. (1971): *Handbook of Physical Medicine and Rehabilitation*. Saunders, Philadelphia.

7. McRae, L. P., and Kartchner, M. M. (1982): Oculoplethysmography. In: *Practical Non-Invasive Vascular Diagnosis 1982*, edited by R. F. Kempczinski and J. S. T. Yao, pp. 181–202. Year Book, Chicago.

8. Meyer, J. S. (1982): Stroke (vascular disease of the brain). In: *Better Homes and Gardens New Family Medical Guide*, edited by E. Keister Jr., pp. 237–247. Meredith Corporation, Des Moines.

9. Miller, B. F., and Keane, C. B. (1972): *Encyclopedia and Dictionary of Medicine and Nursing*. Saunders, Philadelphia.

10. O'Brien, E., and O'Malley, K. (1982): *High Blood Pressure*. Martin Dunitz, London.

11. Paushter, D. M., Modic, M. T., Borkowski, G. P., Weinstein, M. A., and Zeman, R. K. (1984): Magnetic resonance, principles and applications. *Med. Clin. North Am.*, 68:5; 1393–1421.

12. Sahs, A. L., and Hartman, E. C., editors (1976): *Fundamentals of Stroke Care*. Department of Health, Education and Welfare, Washington, D.C.

13. Sidney, L., editor (1975): *Stroke and Its Rehabilitation, 1975*. Waverly Press, Baltimore.
14. String, S. T. (1982): Zira oculoplethysmography. In: *Practical Non-Invasive Vascular Diagnosis 1982*, edited by R. F. Kempczinski and J. S. T. Yao, pp. 203–213. Year Book, Chicago.
15. Toole, J. F. (1982): The brain and nervous system. In: *Better Homes and Gardens New Family Medical Guide*, edited by E. Keister Jr., pp. 189–219. Meredith Corporation, Des Moines.
16. Toole, J. F. (1984): *Cerebrovascular Disorders*, 3rd ed. Raven Press, New York.
17. Winter, C. C., and Barker, M. R. (1972): *Nursing Care of Patients with Urological Diseases*. Mosby, St. Louis.

BOOKLETS

1. *After Your Stroke*. North Carolina Baptist Hospital Educational Department, Winston-Salem, 1982.
2. *Aphasia and the Family*. American Heart Association, Dallas, 1969.
3. *Comfortably Yours—Aids for Easier Living*. Comfortably Yours, Maywood, New Jersey, 1986.
4. Crater, N. N. (1981): *Bladder Training and Self Catheterization*. North Carolina Baptist Hospital Education Department, Winston-Salem.
5. Dawns, J. B. (1973): *Skin Care, Patient Teaching Guide*. Woodrow Wilson Rehabilitation Center, Fishersville, Virginia.
6. *Essentials of the Neurological Examination*. SmithKline Corporation, Philadelphia, 1974.
7. *For Men Only: The Basic Facts About Urinary Incontinence*. Cheesebrough-Ponds, Hospital Products Division, Greenwich, Connecticut, 1970.
8. *Home Health Care Specialog*. Sears Roebuck, Chicago, 1986.

9. Lavin, J. (1985): *There Is Sex After Stroke, Be Stroke Smart*. National Stroke Association, Denver.

10. *Magnetic Resonance Imaging*. Picker, Highland Heights, Ohio.

11. McHenry, L. C., Jr. (1980): *Essentials of Stroke Diagnosis and Management*. SmithKline Corporation, Philadelphia.

12. *1986 Stroke Facts*. American Heart Association, Dallas, 1985.

13. Schaefer, S. (1985): *Bladder Problems Following Stroke, Be Stroke Smart*. National Stroke Association, Denver.

14. Sex counseling for handicapped persons—an avenue toward intimacy. *Rehabil. Brief*, 1(13), 1978.

15. Smith, F. A. (1980): *After Your Stroke*. North Carolina Baptist Hospital Patient Education Department, Winston-Salem.

16. *A Source Book: Rehabilitating the Person with Spinal Cord Injuries—The Neurogenic Bladder*. Veterans Administration, Washington, D.C.

17. *Stroke—Hope Through Research*. U.S. Department of Health and Human Services, National Institutes of Health, Bethesda, 1983.

18. *Stroke: Why Do They Behave That Way?* American Heart Association, Dallas, 1975.

19. *Strokes—A Guide for the Family*. American Heart Association, Dallas, 1981.

20. Talley, C. (1982): *Bladder Management of Stroke Patient*. Forsyth Memorial Hospital Regional Rehabilitation Center, Winston-Salem.

21. Wilcox, N. G. (1984): *Skin Care*. North Carolina Baptist Hospital Acute Rehabilitation, Winston-Salem.

Glossary

Activities of daily living Self-care skills, such as feeding, bathing, and dressing.

Amaurosis fugax Sudden fleeting loss of vision in an entire eye.

Aneurysm A weakened area in the wall of an artery that stretches and enlarges to form a balloon when filled with blood. An aneurysm is not dangerous unless it ruptures or bursts.

Anticoagulants Drugs given to inhibit the blood clotting mechanism by keeping the blood in a fluid state and preventing abnormal clotting.

Antiplatelet agents Drugs that have a destructive action on blood platelets.

Aphasia Disturbance or loss of ability to express or comprehend spoken or written language.

Apraxia Loss of ability to carry out purposeful movements or use an object correctly.

Arteriosclerosis Thickening of the walls of an artery resulting in a loss of the ability of the artery to stretch. More commonly referred to as hardening of the arteries.

Arteriovenous malformation (AVM) Abnormality of blood vessels in the brain in which there is an abnormal communication between the arterial and venous systems.

Arteritis Inflammation of an artery.

Atherosclerosis A form of arteriosclerosis in which the inside walls of the artery become thick owing to a buildup of deposits of fat and cholesterol. This buildup causes the inside of the artery to become narrowed, thereby decreasing the flow of blood through it.

Bruit Abnormal sound noted while listening with a stethoscope to areas that supply blood. It indicates a disturbance in blood flow.

203

Cerebral angiography/arteriography X-ray films of an artery obtained with the use of an opaque dye injected into the bloodstream. These tests are useful for noting areas of blood vessel narrowing or obstruction.

Cerebrovascular accident (CVA) Also referred to as cerebral vascular accident, apoplexy, stroke, or cerebral infarction. It results in defects in the functioning of the brain due to interruption of its blood supply.

Cognition Awareness.

Contractures Loss of motion of a joint caused by a shortened muscle or tendon.

Coordination Ability to control movements smoothly.

Credé's maneuver Downward pushing on the area over the bladder.

Dysarthria Imperfect articulation of speech, often expressed as slurring.

Dysphagia Difficulty when swallowing.

Dysphasia Impairment of the ability to comprehend and express spoken or written language.

Embolus Blood clot or piece of cholesterol or fat that lodges in arteries too small for it to pass through, thereby preventing blood from reaching areas beyond the obstruction.

Endarterectomy Excision of thickened areas in the arteries that are due to plaque buildup on the artery wall.

Epidural hemorrhage Bleeding that occurs above the outer hard covering of the brain.

Extension Straightening out a joint.

Flexion Bending a joint.

Frequency Increased number of times of urination.

Hemiparesis Muscular weakness of one side of the body.

Hemiplegia Paralysis of one side of the body.

Homonymous hemianopsia Loss of one-half of the visual field on the outer (temporal) side of one eye and one-half of the field on the inner (nasal) side of the corresponding eye.

Hypersensitivity Increased awareness of touch.

Incontinence Inability to control the passage of urine or feces.

Lumen The cavity or channel within an artery or vein.

Metabolism Sum of the processes in the building up and breaking down of tissues in the body.

Myocardial infarction Commonly referred to as a heart attack. It results from death of heart muscle tissue.

Nocturia Increased urination at night.

Occupational therapy Treatment using purposeful activity to reduce or overcome physical disabilities; works with self-care skills and activities of daily living.

Perseveration Persistence of one reply or idea.

Physical therapy Treatment to increase muscle strength, coordination, and endurance in an effort to improve independence and function.

Plaque Fat and cholesterol deposits adhering to the artery wall.

Quad cane Four-pronged cane.

Range of motion Exercises used to keep a joint from getting stiff.

Reflux Backflow of urine into the kidneys.

Residual Urine left in the bladder.

Retention Inability to empty the bladder.

Reversible ischemic neurological deficit (RIND) Symptoms of neurological deficits that resolve within weeks.

Sensorimotor Both sensory and motor (sensations and movements).

Splints A plastic support used to position body parts.

Subarachnoid hemorrhage Bleeding that occurs under a thin membrane that covers the brain. Usually results from an aneurysm bursting.

Subdural hemorrhage Hemorrhage under the outer hard covering of the brain. Usually results from the head striking an immovable object.

Thrombosis Formation of blood clots inside a blood vessel.

Transfer To move from one surface to another: for instance, moving from the bed to a wheelchair.

Transient global amnesia   Loss of memory lasting minutes to hours and resolving within 24 hours.

Transient ischemic attack (TIA)   Episode of neurological deficit that generally lasts a few minutes and resolves within 24 hours. Often referred to as a warning sign of a stroke.

Urgency   Increased need to urinate.

Subject Index